WOMEN PIONEERS
OF MEDICAL RESEARCH

WOMEN PIONEERS OF MEDICAL RESEARCH

Biographies of 25 Outstanding Scientists

King-Thom Chung

Foreword by Hubert A. Lechevalier

McFarland & Company, Inc., Publishers

Jefferson, North Carolina, and London

LIBRARY OF CONGRESS CATALOGUING-IN-PUBLICATION DATA

Chung, King-Thom, 1943–
    Women pioneers of medical research : biographies of 25
outstanding scientists / King-Thom Chung ; foreword by
Hubert A. Lechevalier.
        p.   cm.
    Includes bibliographical references and index.

    ISBN 978-0-7864-2927-1
    softcover : 50# alkaline paper ∞

    1. Medicine — Research.   2. Biology — Research.   3. Women
scientists — Biography.   4. Scientists — Biography.   5. Medicine —
History.   I. Title.
[DNLM: 1. Biomedical Research — Biography.   2. Biomedical
Research — history.   3. History, Modern 1601– .   4. Women —
Biography.   WZ150C559w   2010]
R850.C485   2010
610.72 — dc22   2009040830

British Library cataloguing data are available

On the cover: from top left Lady Mary Wortley Montagu; radium electron
shell; nystatin formula; Florence Nightingale (all Wikimedia Commons);
Elizabeth Blackwell (©2010 clipart.com)

Manufactured in the United States of America

McFarland & Company, Inc., Publishers
    Box 611, Jefferson, North Carolina 28640
    www.mcfarlandpub.com

TABLE OF CONTENTS

ACKNOWLEDGMENTS

I am greatly indebted to the late Dr. Cornelius B. Van Niel (1897–1985) for his personal inspiration and encouragement for my academic development. Thanks to his recommendation, I had the opportunity to complete my doctoral degree under the guidance of the renowned late Dr. Robert E. Hungate (1906–2004) of the University of California, Davis. Through many years of their mentorships, I learned the importance of the human side of science. Without their influence, I would never have had the idea of writing this book.

I am also especially appreciative of the late Dr. Deam H. Ferris (1912–1993) for his generous help in making this book possible. Initially, I didn't plan to write biographies until I retired from active research and teaching. At Deam's insistence, I began writing as early as possible in 1989. Deam generously edited some of my earlier writings. Unfortunately, he passed away in December of 1993, but without Deam's encouragement, this book would probably still be in its infancy. Deam felt strongly about the importance of the human side of science and encouraged me greatly to write this book.

Also, special appreciation goes to Dr. Hubert Lechevalier, Professor Emeritus, Rutgers University, who generously offered many good suggestions on the content. Thanks also go to Dr. Joan W. Bennett of Rutgers University and Dr. Christien Mortelmans of SRI International for their encouragement and help in publishing some of my biographical articles in journals.

FOREWORD BY
HUBERT A. LECHEVALIER

Dr. King-Thom Chung, a man of indefatigable industry, is not only a teacher and a research microbiologist, but is also one of these rare active scientists with a keen interest in the history of science. In this domain, he focuses on the lives of the scientists. He has written more than 60 short, highly readable biographies of microbiologists where he stresses their dedication to science and to the betterment of mankind.

Women throughout history have displayed as much such dedication as men — and often had to work harder to even be allowed to pursue their passions. As a rule, to succeed, women have to fight conscious or unconscious discrimination. Thus, everything else being equal, their successes are more remarkable than those of men. This is well illustrated in the 25 biographies that constitute this book.

At first glance, it would seem logical that women should practice medicine. From time immemorial, mothers have taken care of their sick children and husbands. We can certainly conclude that women have been in the nursing business for as long as humanity has existed. The next logical steps for women were to be midwives, then physicians specializing in women's diseases and finally expanding their services without gender restriction. We are reaching this last stage, but in this progression there were some backward steps.

There were women physicians in ancient Greece, Rome, and the Byzantine Empire but, although some achieved high social standing, there was already some discrimination against them. For example, in a hospital in Byzantium (Istanbul) there was a ward with three physicians, two men and one women, and (guess what?) the woman doctor was paid half as much as the male doctors (Parker, 1997).

In the early Middle Ages, in Europe, there were no special efforts to prevent women from practicing medicine, and many had excellent reputations as healers. But when an effort was made to protect the public from charlatans by requiring that physicians be certified or show proof of medical school attendance, women faced a serious problem, for most universities did not admit female students. Even if they had graduated from a university, women's problems were not over. They could be accused of being witches or, as pre-

1

scribed in a statute passed in Valencia in 1239, they could be "whipped through the town" (Solomon, 1997).

Fortunately, the prosecution of women accused of practicing medicine illegally was not always a great public relations success. In Paris, in 1322, Jacqueline Félicie de Almania defended herself by producing as witnesses some of her patients, who testified that they had been cured by Jacqueline after some of the renowned (male) authorities of the time had shown themselves to be totally ineffective (Solomon, 1997).

Reluctantly, little by little, medical schools opened their doors to women. In Berlin, this took place in 1908, but individual professors could still exclude women from their courses. One of the reasons offered for keeping women out of the classrooms was that they distracted the male students — to the point that, in Leipzig, a romantic medical student was supposedly so disturbed by the charms of a Russian female student that he committed suicide. Effectively, Czarist Russia was a pioneer in the field of female education, not only opening the medical schools to women but also fully funding their studies. By 1914, women formed 10 percent of the Russian medical profession. This trend continued under the communist regime and by 1967, 70 percent of Russian physicians were women (Meyer, 1977). By contrast, in 1970 only 7.2 percent of American physicians were women (Walsh, 1977). In the year 2000, the prediction, based on medical school enrollments, was that by the first third of the 21st century 40 percent of American physicians will be women (Morantz-Sanchez, 2000).

In England, the University of London opened all degrees to women in 1878. An examination of England's Registry of Medical Women from 1882 reveals that the handful of women listed with a M.D. degree had all been educated on the continent with the exception of Elizabeth Blackwell, who received her degree in America in 1858 (Blake, 1990).

Of course not all the women who contributed to advance in medicine were physicians. Madame Curie, for example, was a physicist. This does not mean that women scientists who were not physicians were much better received by their colleagues than those who wanted to practice medicine. Far too often, these great scientists were treated unfairly and not accorded the respect they deserved. Dr. Chung's book tells us the stories of 25 women who persevered against such discrimination in order to pursue their dreams. All humankind has benefited from that perseverance.

Further Reading

Blake, C. *The Charge of the Parasols.* London: Women's Press, 1990.
Meyer, P. They met in Zürich: nineteenth-century German and Russian women physicians.

In *Women Healers and Physicians: Climbing a Long Hill.* Edited by L. R. Furst. Lexington: University Press of Kentucky, 1997. 151–177.

Morantz-Sanchez, R. *Sympathy and Science: Women Physicians in American Medicine.* Chapel Hill: University of North Carolina Press, 2000.

Parker, H. N. Women doctors in Greece, Rome, and the Byzantine Empire. In *Women Healers and Physicians: Climbing a Long Hill.* Edited by L. R. Furst. Lexington: University Press of Kentucky, 1997. 131–150.

Solomon, M. Women healers and the power to disease in late medieval Spain. In *Women Healers and Physicians: Climbing a Long Hill.* Edited by L. R. Furst. Lexington: University Press of Kentucky, 1997. 79–92.

Walsh, M. R. *"Doctors Wanted: No Women Need Apply": Sexual Barriers in the Medical Profession, 1835–1975.* New Haven: Yale University Press, 1977.

Hubert A. Lechevalier, professor of microbiology at Rutgers University, 1951–1991, was a visiting investigator at the Academy of Sciences of the Soviet Union (1958–1959) and at the Pasteur Institute in Paris (1961–1962). A researcher in actinomycetes and their products, he is the codiscoverer of such antibiotics as neomycin and candicidin, and the coauthor of Three Centuries of Microbiology.

PREFACE

We often take for granted our longevity, enjoyment of modern conveniences, and superior medical care as simply a part of our life. But modern civilization as we know it today has emerged largely within the last century and a half. Our standard of living, which is beyond anything our ancestors could have known, is possible because of the hard work and even suffering of the pioneer scientists who made important discoveries and innovations. Life science is a major building block of modern sciences. Even those who are immersed in modern life science research may not know how this knowledge has been accumulated. Much of it was acquired by pioneer scientists including women researchers. Those pioneer investigators are often unknown to the general public and even to many students in the field of life science. The stories of these pioneers have not been told in general textbooks, and are often a neglected subject in literature and history books.

Busy with our daily lives and routines, most of us never think of these researchers. But their stories need to be told, especially for the benefit of our young people who need to understand how our civilization was developed. They also need to know the human values and the creative thinking that brought about such ingenious and marvelous results. I hope that the stories of these researchers will inspire all who read them, especially those young minds looking for guidance. The same challenges that stimulated Florence Nightingale (1820–1910), Elizabeth Blackwell (1821–1910), or Gertrude Elion (1918–1999) can inspire young minds to creativity and further contribute to human civilization.

For this reason, I am interested in the life stories of scientific pioneers. But "pioneering," breaking new ground, moving out into the unknown, is not limited to the past two centuries. The beginnings of a science are memorable, and we can never do too much to honor those who struggled against great odds to lay its foundation, especially when they did so in response to great human need and under great difficulties.

But every era in the history of science has had its share of pioneering, and in this book, the author will explore the life experiences of those who are considered major pioneers in medical science. I have chosen to focus on women scientists because they have been largely ignored. Their life experiences were particularly interesting since many of them often had to struggle against gender bias. Many of them were never given equal opportunities because they had to fight against gender discrimination. Some of their scientific accomplishments did not receive due recognition because of their gender. Their stories are even more inspiring when we see that their astonishing successes were accomplished in unsupportive environments.

In this book I sketch the lives of 25 women pioneers. I specifically chose those in medical research since their work is within my expertise and very specifically touches my mind. You will find that their stories are not only interesting but also inspiring.

Carl Gustav Jung (1875–1961), a founder of modern psychiatry, climaxed his great career by writing a small book summarizing his findings: *The Undiscovered Self.* This book you are reading now might similarly be subtitled: *Medical Science—The Undiscovered Side.*

What is the undiscovered side of science? The human side. While in the laboratory, we are making new technical discoveries, which are important to the progress of society. These new technical discoveries are announced every day in scientific journals, but they often appear to be too technical, usually impersonal and dull. To the initiated students, of course, they may be highly interesting, but to most of us something important is still missing: the human factors that have guided the scientist.

From many years of teaching an introductory course of microbiology to students in health fields, I have found that students seem to draw the most inspiration from lectures that include some stories of the human side of pioneer researchers. A large portion of students in my classes are female students with the aim of entering the fields of medicine or nursing. It seems natural that women pioneers should be among their role models. Who were those pioneer researchers involved in significant discoveries? What were those scientists thinking? What problems did they face? What were their family backgrounds? What were their personal lives? What were the driving forces in their lives? What else did they do besides work in science? The author feels that knowledge of the human side of scientists is as important and as interesting as the scientific side of their work.

New discoveries are still being made today. Let us remember that discoveries have been and are being made by human beings. The life experiences of those pioneer scientists provide us with an in-depth inspiration to learning and creating. They will teach us not only the technical knowledge they have uncovered, which benefits us immensely, but also the value of searching for truth. These are treasures that we can share. After all, humanity is as important as science. This book was written in the spirit of honoring the memory of each pioneer.

During this writing, I have made it a point to note the dates of all significant events involved in the development of each scientist and her research. I have also, in an appendix, included brief biographies of important persons mentioned in the life of each pioneer, so the type of persons they encountered in their professional lives can be seen in a vivid way. After all, each individual story is a part of the history of science. Reading the story of each scientist involves a comprehension of the history in her time and the persons involved during each episode.

The choice of women covered was unavoidably subjective, relying on a combination of an individual's contributions to medical science, the amount of biographical information my research could uncover, and in some cases a particularly compelling life story. The subjects are arranged chronologically. This book, written in the spirit of honoring the memory of each pioneer, represents an attempt to discover and publicize the work of these women to whom we owe a great deal.

King-Thom Chung
The University of Memphis
November 2009

1

MARY WORTLEY MONTAGU (1689–1762)

Promoter of Inoculation Against Smallpox

A woman really virtuous, in the utmost of this expression, has virtue of a purer kind than any philosopher has ever shown; since she knows, if she has sense, and without it there can be no virtue, that mankind is too much prejudiced against her sex, to give her any degree of that fame which is so sharp a spur to any of their great actions. I have some thoughts of exhibiting a set of pictures of such meritorious ladies, where I shall say nothing of the fire of their eyes, or the pureness of their complexions, but give them such praises as befit a rational sensible being: virtues of choice, and not beauties of accident.

The variola (smallpox) virus has killed millions of people through the centuries. The virus probably evolved from an orthopox virus in Africa. It is likely that Egyptian armies were responsible for moving the disease to the Middle East. In A.D. 166, Roman soldiers brought smallpox to Europe where it killed up to 200 people a day. In A.D. 900, the Persian physician Rhazes (860–923 or A.D. 932) recognized smallpox and measles as two distinctly different diseases. Over the centuries, smallpox became the leading infectious disease and epidemic ravaged the world.

European colonization brought smallpox to the Americans and to Africans south of the Sahara. The Spanish conquests of Amerindians in the 16th century coincided with epidemics of smallpox that reduced the Amerindian populations so they were unable to resist the armies of Hernando Cortés and Francisco Pizarro. In 1721, 5,759 cases of smallpox were reported in Boston (population 10,700) and one out of every seven patients died. By the 18th century, smallpox killed 200,000 to 600,000 people every year in Europe.

The physical effect of this disease was devastating. Transmitted through the respiratory route, the virus infected internal organs before being transported through the blood to the skin. Viral growth in the epidermis caused small bumps on the face, upper body, and arms. Over several days the bumps filled with fluid, became inflamed, broke, and formed a soft yellow crust. Blisters of pus and running sores would form, often together with red rashes on the body. In bad cases, the pustules would cover the whole body and form scabs, which would turn to deeply ugly scars.

In the Eastern countries, this disease was equally dreadful, although we have no record of the death toll. But there was great human misery. In China, smallpox was first reported in the first century. Over many centuries, Chinese physicians developed techniques to prevent smallpox. Old Chinese writings dating from the Sung Dynasty (960–1280) describe the technique known as variolation, also called inoculation. This was done by removing scabs from drying pustules of a patient suffering from a mild case of smallpox, grinding the scabs to a fine powder, and inserting the powder into the nose of the person to be protected. Such an inoculated person would usually develop a mild case of smallpox and eventually develop immunity to it. Because one of the early kings of the Q'ing Dynasty (1644–1911), Shuen Chi (1644–1662), died of smallpox, this method of prevention was widely practiced among the royal soldiers of the Q'ing Empire in the 17th century in China. The basic concept of the Chinese physicians was "poison against poison." Although the concept of immunity was not developed at that time, the method worked effectively and saved millions. In 1688, Russian doctors were sent to Beijing to learn the technique of "humanpox inoculation" from the Chinese with the result that this method of smallpox prevention was also practiced in Russia. A similar method of prevention was practiced in Turkey, where smallpox was rampant. Although we do not have direct evidence to prove the origin of this method, it is likely that China was the original inventor of this technique and introduced it into Turkey.

In Turkey, preventive methods were usually exercised in the late summer by a group of elderly women. Each woman would carry in a nutshell a small sample of pus that had been collected from patients with mild cases of smallpox. With a large needle, the woman would quickly scratch open a vein on the limb of one of her "customers." The woman would then dip her needle into the pus in the nutshell and smear it on the open vein, covering the wound with a piece of nutshell and binding it. The inoculated patients would develop a mild case of fever and immunity to smallpox.

Communication between the East and the West was rare, especially in medicine. The practice of Turkey's preventive medicine for smallpox was not noticed by the West until the early 18th century. This practice was introduced to the West by Lady Mary Wortley Montagu, a woman of letters. She was not a medical doctor; yet because of her introduction of this inoculation technique, a revolution in medicine slowly took place, leading to the emergence of modern microbiology and immunology. It is worthwhile to learn a little about the life of this unusual woman who was considered a "scientific lady" by some writers. She was also an important feminist writer of the 18th century.

Lady Mary was born in 1689 to an affluent family. Her father was Evelyn Pierrepoint, the fifth Earl and first Duke of Kingston, a Yorkshire gentleman. Her mother was Lady Mary Fielding. Mary was the niece of the famous novelist Henry Fielding (1707–1754). Her mother died when she was only four years old, and her father took little interest in his family. Little Mary was a gifted child and made good use of her father's extensive library to educate herself. Bishop Gilbert Burnet of Salisbury (1643–1715) was one of her mentors. She began writing poems and an autobiography at an early age. Young Mary was fascinated by literature. She determined to read Ovid in the original. She would take a Latin grammar book and dictionary from the family library and hide with them for several hours a day. She became very good in Latin. Later, her father was so pleased with her self-learning that he arranged to have her tutored in Italian. She also learned French and later Turkish. At age 20, Lady Mary sent Bishop Burnet her English translation of the first-century Greek Stoic philosopher Epictetus (c.55–c.135).

Lady Mary was an active feminist, well liberated at least 300 years ahead of her time. She secured her own liberation by virtue of her innate intelligence and self-education. Her speaking tone was described as like a viper and her pen like a razor. She could make her presence felt in any society. She intended to experience life to the fullest and left an account of that life in diaries and letters. In a letter she sent to Bishop Burnet, she wrote: "My sex is usually forbidden studies of this nature —. We are permitted no books but such as tend to the weakening and effeminating of the mind."

Mary was good in literature, and she was able to quote a poem of Quintus Horatus Horace (65–8 B.C.) that attracted the attention of Edward Wortley Montagu, who believed that women should be literate and educated. The two fell in love. In 1712, in order to avoid an arranged marriage, Mary eloped to Constantinople with Montagu, who was a Whig member of Parliament. Their son, Edward, Jr., was born in 1713. In 1717, Montagu became the new English ambassador in Constantinople, at the court of the Ottoman Empire. Mary and the child Edward, Jr., accompanied him to Constantinople. A daughter, Mary, was born in 1717.

In Turkey, Lady Mary did not spend most of her time inside the Embassy building. She was interested in Turkey's culture, particularly concerning women's rights, and found the Turks interesting. She was quick to observe and record political and social customs of which she approved. She noticed their justice regarding married women's property rights in Turkey; in particular she noted Turkish women's right in divorce to keep their own money and also receive maintenance from the husband.

She was also interested in matters of health and medicine, probably partly because her brother had died of smallpox. Because Lady Mary herself had suffered a mild case of smallpox in her own life, she knew that she could observe the disease from close quarters with little fear. She made a detailed record of what she saw in Constantinople about smallpox and the local method of inoculation, which she called "engrafting." In April of 1717, she wrote a letter to her friend Sarah Chiswell giving the details of the inoculation procedure. She wrote: "The smallpox, so fatal, and so general among us, is here entirely harmless by the invention of *Engrafting*— the old woman comes with a nutshell full of the matter of the best sort of smallpox ... and puts into the vein as much venom as can lie upon the head of her needle.... There is no example of any one that has died in it; and you may believe I am very satisfied of the safety of the experiment, since I intend to try it on my little son." She arranged for her son Edward to be inoculated sometime in 1718. Edward was the first recorded Englishman to experience this form of inoculation against smallpox. He survived. Since smallpox was so common in Europe, Lady Montagu considered it nothing short of her patriotic duty to make "this useful invention" fashionable in England.

After returning to England in 1721, she had her daughter, Mary (who later became Lady Bute), inoculated for smallpox. She patronized Dr. Charles Maitland, who had been a physician to the English mission during her stay in Constantinople, and persuaded him to begin to practice inoculation. This practice immediately came under serious attack by the medical profession and even the Church. But Lady Montagu was determined to further her goal: the widespread inoculation of the population of England against smallpox. She went directly to the court of King George I (1660–1727) with whom Lady Montagu had good contacts. She was able to interest Caroline, the Princess of Wales. Through the good offices of the court, and with the help of the very distinguished secretary of the Royal Society, Sir Hans Sloane (1660–1753), she arranged a series of perhaps the most unusual medical experiments that had ever been conducted by men or women. Seven condemned criminals from Newgate prison were given the option of submitting to the gallows or to Lady Montagu's newly imported smallpox inoculation. The criminals chose inoculation. They survived to be free with nothing worse than their inoculation scars.

The experiment was repeated on half a dozen orphan children. Again, they all survived. In 1722 King George I was sufficiently impressed by Lady Montagu's successes to be persuaded to have two of his grandchildren inoculated. This was also successful. Many English people followed this practice, and consequently, it spread rapidly throughout England, continental Europe, and North America. Lady Montagu became a celebrity in her own time and her name entered medical history in addition to literary history. She declared sweepingly, "I know nobody that has hitherto repented of the operation."

Variolation was not perfect. Two or three percent of the inoculations resulted in fatalities. But the number of deaths was far outnumbered by the lives saved. Variolation continued to be practiced until the introduction of cowpox vaccine developed by Edward Jenner (1749–1823) at the end of the 18th century.

Lady Montagu was extremely intelligent, witty, and beautiful. She would always be at the center of intellectual society. She surrounded herself with the intellectual company of literary and scientific individuals at her salon at Twickenham. Her salon included scientists, the poet Alexander Pope (1688–1744), John Gay (1685–1732), and numerous other famous intellectuals. She wrote poems as well as one play titled *Essays and Poems and Simplicity, a Comedy.* She was also a member of the Bluestocking Society, a salon of scientists and intellectuals, whose name derived from the clothing first sported at club meetings by botanist Benjamin Stillingfleet (1702–1771). Unfortunately, "bluestocking" later became a derogatory label aimed at women intellectuals.

Lady Montagu was truly a liberated woman. In 1736, at the age of 47, she fell in love with a 24-year-old Italian, Francesco Algarotti. She left her husband to move to Italy in order to be with Algarotti in 1739. Algarotti was the author of a popular book for women on Newtonian science. Although Algarotti later moved to the court of Frederick the Great in Berlin, Lady Montagu decided to stay in Italy and make it her home. She settled in Venice and reestablished her salon on the Grand Canal of Venice. She enjoyed Italian culture because she felt it was more accepting of women scholars, writers, and scientists. She produced many writings while she stayed in Italy. Some of her enduring writings are her letters that concerned the education of her oldest granddaughter, Mary Bute.

Lady Montagu returned to England following her husband's death in 1761. She died of breast cancer in 1762. Lady Montagu's relationship with her son, Edward, Jr. (1713–1776), was rather unfortunate. Edward, Jr., was a troublesome child. Mary's daughter married Lord Bute, who became King George III's right hand man. Dr. Rebecca Craighill Lancefield (1895–1981), a great microbiologist who did famous work on the serological classification of streptococci, was one of Lady Montagu's descendents.

*   *   *

Lady Montagu's fame came more from her brilliant writings, extraordinary lifestyle, and uncompromising feminism than from her important work on variolation. Many of the negative comments about Mary Montagu came from Alexander Pope, a poet and writer. Pope was in love with her and wrote a number of poems dedicated to her. When Pope openly declared his love to her in 1722, Mary refused and laughed, leading Pope to become her enemy and attack her via literature. Pope's attacks were harmful, damaging the career and social standing of her husband, a member of Parliament. Although she attempted to help her husband's political party by publishing a newspaper called *The Nonsense of Common-sense* against the popular Opposition paper *Common-Sense*, their marriage was not successful, although no divorce was formally reported.

Lady Mary Montagu was not a trained scientist. She probably never touched a microscope in her life. Her observation of smallpox inoculation was far from original even in England. A similar form of inoculation was probably in existence in some parts of Britain — in Scotland and Wales — when she introduced it as a novelty to England. But she had applied certain scientific principles to her observation. She had "thought through" and formed a theory linking inoculation with mild smallpox to immunity from dangerous smallpox. She also had devised unusual experiments to test her theory, experiments unimaginable in her time. But she had her own children vaccinated before she tried it on others. She had also published her results with fanfare. Today we call this publicity. She certainly deserves great credit for the development of variolation, which led to Edward Jenner's work with cowpox and also to the germ theory of Louis Pasteur (1822–1895) and Robert Koch (1843–1910). Lady Montagu's work demonstrated a fruitful interaction between the East and West and was one step in bringing human civilization to a new stage of better health.

Further Reading

Case, C. L., and K.-T. Chung. 1997. Montagu and Jenner: The campaign against smallpox. *SIM News* 47: 58–60.

Nester, Eugene W., D. G. Anderson, C. E. Roberts, Jr., N. N. Pearsall, and M. T. Nester. 2001. *Microbiology: A Human Perspective*. 3rd ed. New York: McGraw-Hill. 413.

Reid, R. 1975. *Microbes and Men*. New York: Saturday Review Press. 9–14.

Szpir, M. 1993. No stock in smallpox virus? *American Scientist* **81**: 526–527.

Tortora, G. J., B. R. Funke, and C. L. Case. 2003. *Microbiology: An Introduction*. 8th ed. San Francisco: Benjamin Cummings Pearson. 600–601.

Selected Writings by Lady Montagu

1. *Essays and Poems and Simplicity, a Comedy.* 1993. Edited by Robert Halsband and Isobel Grundy. Oxford: Clarendon.

2. *The Letters and Works.* (1861.) 1886–1908. Edited by Lord Wharncliffe and W. Moy Thomas. 2 vols. 3rd ed. Reprint, London: George Bell.

2

FLORENCE NIGHTINGALE
(1820–1910)

Founder of Modern Nursing

Florence Nightingale is well known as the founder of modern nursing. She raised nursing to a respectable professional level. In the early 1800s, nursing was not a profession in England. Nurses were drawn from the lowest social classes and were not educated. Therefore, they were not respectable in those days. Nightingale was able to change that impression. She developed a new dimension in nursing and revolutionized the education system for nurses. She raised the nursing standard and made nursing an important part of modern medicine, which affected human health profoundly. She also pioneered the use of statistical approaches for medical studies and improved the health measures both for military hospitals and the general public. She was also a pioneer epidemiologist.

Florence was born on May 12, 1820, in the city of Florence, Italy, to an affluent family. Her father was William Edward Nightingale (1794–1874), a Cambridge-educated intellectual, and her mother was Frances Smith Nightingale (1794–1874). Florence had an elder sister, Parthenope (1818–1890), who was born in Naples, where their parents were on their honeymoon. Her family moved back to London when Florence was age two. Extremely wealthy English landowners, they had two homes. One was Lea Hurst in Derbyshire, where they spent their summer months. The other was Embley Park in Hampshire, where they spent their winter months. Lea Hurst now is a retirement home, and Embley Park is now a school. The family socialized in the highest circles of London and became very influential.

In those days in England, like most places in the world, women did not typically attend school or pursue professional careers. Their purposes in life were to marry and bear children. However, Mr. Nightingale was an enlightened man and believed that women should be educated. He personally taught both Florence and Parthenope Italian, Latin, Greek, philosophy, history, writing, and mathematics.

Florence was a very attractive young woman who had many suitors. However, she believed that marriage could never satisfy her ambitions. She considered that conventional marriage would be like suicide. She turned down marriage proposals from rich young pursuers. She was clearly determined to be a single woman.

Florence believed strongly in God. It was said that she heard the voice of God in her garden in 1837, which she described as a calling to do God's work. Because of her religious belief, she had a conviction that the best way to serve God was through service to mankind.

To the astonishment of her parents, Florence was interested in a career in nursing. To pursue any career was radical thinking for a woman of Nightingale's social class. Nurses in those days were uneducated and untrained, and their behaviors were not admirable. They had a reputation for rudeness and even promiscuity. Florence herself told her father that she had been informed by the head nurse in a London hospital that she "had never known a nurse who was not drunk." Florence's father hoped that she would change her mind, get married, and settle down.

When her parents forbade her to take up nursing, she turned more toward God for guidance. Florence's conviction to the service of God through taking care of patients was stronger than ever. She felt that her mission in life was to develop a new style of nursing. She read voraciously about medicine and health care, spent some time inspecting hospitals in London, and worked privately with children of the slums. During that period of her life, we can well imagine her frustration and discouragement, but also her determination.

While Florence was in conflict with her parents' wishes, it was decided that she would tour Europe with their family friends Charles and Selina Bracebridge. The three traveled to Italy, Egypt, and Greece, returning in July 1850 through Germany. In Germany, they visited Pastor Theodore Fliedner's hospital and school for deaconesses at Kaiserwerth, near Dusseldorf. In 1851 she was able to persuade her parents to allow her to return to Kaiserwerth and spend three months at Fliedner's hospital. The hospital was later called Institute Protestant Deaconesses, Kaiserwerth. Later, against the will of her parents, she served as an apprentice at another hospital operated by the Sisters of Mercy in St. Germain, near Paris. At this stage of her life, she was able to start out in her beloved profession.

With the training and experience as a nurse, Florence returned to London in 1853. Soon she got her first job as an unpaid superintendent of London's Establishment for Gentlewomen During Illness. Her job was to supervise the nurses, to implement the functioning of the physical plant, and to guarantee the purity of the medicines. She successfully improved the institution, and it became the best of the time, open to patients of all classes and religions. However, her desire to establish a formal training school for nurses had not yet materialized.

In 1854 a war broke out between Turkey and Russia. Both England and France entered the war. In September 1854, British and French troops invaded the Crimea, on the north coast of the Black Sea, in support of Turkey in its dispute with Russia. The allied English and French forces scored a quick victory at the Battle of the Alma River on September 20 and began the siege of the Russian naval base at Sevastopol. During this time, the news correspondent of *The Times*, Mr. William Howard Russell, reported that the British Army was decimated by epidemics of cholera and typhus. The sick and wounded British soldiers were left to die without medical attention. There were too few surgeons and not even linen to make bandages. There was not a single qualified nurse in the British military hospital at Scutari near Constantinopole. Their military hospitals were filthy, unhygienic, and unequipped. The British Army was nearly destroyed by infections. On the other hand, the French hospitals had 50 Sisters of Mercy to take care of their patients.

At this stage in history, people did not know that some microorganisms in the air and water or on utensils would cause diseases. Fundamental hygiene was generally lacking. Antiseptics and disinfectants were unheard of. The famous Hungarian medical doctor Ignaz P. Semmelweis (1818–1865) was fired by his boss in Budapest in 1848 because he claimed that puerperal fever was caused by dirty hands of physicians. The germ theory of Robert Koch (1842–1910) was not published until 1872. Who would believe that dirty water and filthy facilities were the major sources of microorganisms causing diseases of war-wounded soldiers?

Newsmen kept reporting how horrible the war was and how terrible the situation of military hospitals were. The public opinion turned against the government's decision to continue the British participation in the war. It was a golden opportunity for the strongly service-oriented Nightingale, who wrote a letter to her longtime friend, Sidney Herbert, the secretary of war, asking to volunteer for service in the Crimea. At the same time, Sidney Herbert was already on his way to ask Nightingale to head a team of 38 nurses to take care of the soldiers. In addition to the backing of the government (but not of the Army), she also obtained strong financial support raised by *The Times*. The work in the Crimea and the conditions she saw were to determine her mission for the rest of her life. She was about to change history.

Nightingale arrived at Scutari on November 5, 1854, and found deplorable medical facilities. The hospital barracks were infested with insects and rats, and sewers loaded with filth were underneath the buildings. The wind blew the foul smell up the pipes of numerous open privies into the corridors and overcrowded wards where the sick were lying on straw mats. The canvas sheets were so coarse that the wounded men begged to be left on their blankets. The laundry was done with cold water, which resulted in many linens being so verminous that they had to be destroyed. Essential surgical and medical supplies were lacking, and their distribution was blocked by military red tape. The weak and emaciated patients suffered from frostbite and dysentery as well as from their wounds. The resulting epidemics of cholera and typhus caused the greatest loss of lives at Scutari. The mortality rate at the hospital was 42.7 percent of the cases treated in February of 1855.

In military history the main cause of death in war was disease rather than wounds sustained in battle. According to Nightingale's statistical data, the mortality rate among the troops was 60 percent per annum from disease alone during the first months of the Crimean campaign. This rate of death exceeded that of the Great Plague of 1665 in London. If replacements had not been sent, disease alone would have wiped out the entire British Army in Crimea.

Nightingale showed real skill as an administrator and rose to the challenge to change the situation in the Crimea and establish an effective hospital. However, there was strong resistance from the military authorities. The military men resented the fact that Nightingale's authority was independent of the armed services. At first, her nurses were not even allowed on the wards. She had to struggle against petty officials. For example, in one incident, the supply officer refused to distribute badly needed shirts from his store until the entire shipment could be inspected by an official of the Board of Survey.

Yet Nightingale accomplished what was impossible for others because she was independent from the military and had her private source of funds. She strongly and effectively changed the woefully inadequate situation in the hospital at Scutari. She established her own laundry, including boilers to heat the water. She installed extra kitchens in the hospitals and secured diverse supplies: socks, shirts, knives and forks, wooden spoons, tin baths, cabbage and carrots, operating tables, towels and soap, small-tooth combs, materials for destroying lice, scissors, bed pans, and pillows. In addition to the funds provided by *The Times*, she also received funds from other philanthropists and from her own private funds.

Despite her busy schedule as an administrator, Florence still found time to take care of patients herself. She banned all other women from the wards (some of them had been sent back home because of delinquent behavior). Often at night, she carried a little lamp in her hand to inspect the nursing facilities and to take care of her patients. The famous American poet Henry Wadsworth Longfellow (1807–1882) immortalized this lady with a lamp and wrote in one of his poems in 1857, "Lo! in that house of misery/A lady with a lamp I see." As a result of Nightingale's efforts, half a year after her arrival at Scutari, the mortality rate in the hospital had dropped from 42.7 percent to 2.2 percent.

Nightingale returned to London in July 1856, four months after the end of the Crimean War. By that time, though only 36 years old, she was a world famous figure. Despite the popularity and honors she would receive, she decided that the most appropriate recognition for her services would be the establishment of a commission to investigate military medical care. She wrote that some 9,000 soldiers died from causes that might have been prevented. The tragedy of needless death was continuing in every army barracks and hospital. It could be stopped only by the establishment, throughout the Army Medical Service, of the sanitary reforms that had saved so many lives at Scutari. Nightingale set herself a goal to achieve that.

How could Nightingale convince the authorities to achieve the reform? She saw that the most convincing method was through statistical methods of analyzing data and information and then presenting figures and numbers to the authorities. At Scutari, she collected a tremendous amount of records, especially the number of deaths for establishing an accurate mortality rate that could be compared and analyzed. When Nightingale returned to England, she met Dr. William Farr (1807–1883), a physician and professional statistician. She searched for guidance from Dr. Farr and reorganized the data she had gathered at Scutari. She saw that medical statistics could be used as a tool for improving medical care in military and civilian hospitals. She used various methods to calculate mortality. Nightingale's sanitary reforms began in March 1855. By the end of the Crimean War, the death rate among sick British soldiers in Turkey was not much more than it was among soldiers in England.

She also found that soldiers in England living in barracks were in unhealthy conditions. The mortality rate of soldiers between the age of 20 and 35 who were in England during peace time was nearly twice that of civilians. Clearly, the need for sanitary improvement in the military was not limited to hospitals in the fields. Using her statistical data, she convinced Queen Victoria (1819–1901) and Prince Albert, as well as Prime Minister Lord Palmerston (1784–1865), that there was a need to initiate a formal investigation of military health care and also to establish a Royal Commission on the Health of the Army. The commission was formed in May of 1857. Nightingale actively participated in this investigation and strongly influenced the commission's work. As a result of this inquiry she wrote and published privately an 800-page book titled *Notes on Matters Affecting the Health, Efficiency and Hospital Administration of the British Army.* In this book, she included a section of statistics accompanied by diagrams. Nightingale was a true pioneer in the graphical representation of statistics. She invented polar-area charts in which the statistic being represented is proportional to the area of a wedge in a circular diagram. Dr. William Farr called this book the best publication that was ever written on statistical diagrams.

Nightingale's efforts resulted in the establishment of several sub-commissions to carry out the reforms recommended by the Royal Commission. These included physical alterations to military barracks and hospitals; improvements in ventilation, heating, sewage disposal, water supply, and kitchens; establishing a military medical school; and reorganizing the Army's procedures for gathering medical statistics.

Nightingale also paid a lot of attention to the health of British soldiers in India. In collaboration with Dr. Farr, she studied the sickness and mortality rate of those soldiers. She sent inquiry forms to the various British stations in India for information on sanitary conditions there. Between 1858 and 1859, she lobbied successfully for the establishment of another Royal Commission to look into the problem in India. From this investigation, she found that the death rate among the troops in India was six times higher than the rate among civilians in England. The major causes were poor sewage systems, overcrowding in the barracks, lack of exercise, and inadequate numbers of hospitals. Sanitary reforms were also applied there. In 1873, after 10 years of sanitary reforms, Nightingale reported that the mortality rate among the soldiers in India had declined from 69 to 18 per 1,000.

As we have seen, in addition to being interested in health care reform, Nightingale developed a strong commitment to statistics, which provided an organized way of learning from experience. The statistical data kept by hospitals in Nightingale's time were neither accurate nor uniform. Nightingale thought that uniform and accurate statistics would improve particular methods of treatment and would bring statistical proof of special operations. Consequently, these improvements would lead to medical progress. With the aid of Professor Farr and other physicians, Nightingale developed a Model Hospital Statistical Form that was approved at the International Congress of Statistics held in London in the summer of 1860. The new statistical form provided many advantages and was far ahead of its time. Unfortunately, it was also overly complex, and its idiosyncratic system for the classification of diseases (devised by Dr. Farr) was strongly opposed by many pathologists. As a result of these problems, the form was never put into general use.

Nightingale's commitment to statistics was closely tied to her religious convictions. She was strongly influenced by the theory of Lambert Adolphe-Jacques Quetélet (1796–1874), founder of modern social statistics. She thought that laws governing social phenomena and the laws of moral progress were God's laws to be revealed by statistics. She struggled to get the study of statistics introduced into higher education. Unfortunately, she did not realize that dream in her lifetime.

One of the important persons Nightingale had encountered in her life was Elizabeth Blackwell (1821–1910), America's first female physician. These two women met and corresponded during the 1850s. They discussed the possibility of establishing a program to train women in medicine. However, their goals were entirely different and as a result, each pursued her own direction. Nightingale was interested in establishing a nursing school for women that would promote women's subsidiary role in medicine. Nightingale never thought that women should seek to be physicians. On the other hand, Blackwell and some others were more interested in making women professionally equal with men in the medical field.

Nightingale received many honors. She was the recipient of Order of Merit from King Edward VIII of the United Kingdom in 1907. She was the first woman to receive this award. She was also awarded the Cross of Merit from Germany and Secours aux Blessés Militaires from France.

Nightingale was a very good writer. She published 200 books, reports, and pamphlets. The most well known book was *Notes on Nursing*, which laid down the nursing principles of careful observation and sensitivity to the patient's needs. This book has been translated into eleven foreign languages and is still in use. Other notable books include *Notes on Matters Affecting the Health, Efficiency and Hospital Administration of the British Army*, 1858; *Notes on Hospitals*, 1859; *Life or Death in India*, 1874; and *Notes on the Sanitary States of the Army in India*, 1881. Her writings gave an enormous stimulation to the study of sanitation problems in England and the world.

After Nightingale's return from the Crimea, her health was not good. She was primarily confined to her bedroom. Her poor health might have been related to a fever she contracted in the Crimea, but some suggested that she did not have a physical illness at all; her illness was interpreted by Pickering as psychoneurosis. Nevertheless, she continued to exercise her influence by receiving frequent visitors and by maintaining extensive correspondence. With money from the Nightingale Fund raised by public subscription, she fulfilled her early goal in life and founded the Nightingale School of Nursing at St. Thomas' Hospital and also at King's College Hospital in London in 1860. She also advised and supported William Rathbone in the development of district nursing in Liverpool. Although she did not supervise the schools directly, the training of nurses followed her principles completely. These principles included an insistence that nurses have their technical training in hospitals specially organized for that purpose, and that they live in a home fit to form their moral life and discipline.

Nightingale lived at 10 South Street, Mayfair, in the West End of London from 1865. She occasionally visited Embley, Lea Hurst, and her sister's home, Claydon House. Florence Nightingale died on August 13, 1910, in London at age 90. According to her wishes, she was buried at St Margaret's, East Wellow, near her parents' home, Embley Park in Hampshire.

* * *

Nightingale left a rich legacy to human beings. Her strong religious conviction, persistent efforts, and affluent family background helped her realize her goals. Her sanitary reforms of the hospitals were effective in decreasing the microbial contaminations and infections in the hospitals and elsewhere. Even though Nightingale at first had no knowledge of microbiology, her endeavors were precisely an application of microbiology to human welfare. She believed that infection arose spontaneously in dirty and poorly ventilated places. Today, her sanitation measures are fundamental requirements for any medical facility. Microbiological knowledge is mandatory for all nurses in developed countries. Florence Nightingale's vision has influenced the nature of modern health care.

Further Reading

Cohen, I. B. 1984. Florence Nightingale. *Scientific American* **250**: 128–137.
Monteiro, L. 1984. On separate roads: Florence Nightingale and Elizabeth Blackwell. *Sign* **9**: 540.
Pickering, G. 1974. *Creative Malady*. New York: Dell.

3

ELIZABETH BLACKWELL
(1821–1910)

Champion of Medical Education for Women

*The study and practice of medicine is ... but one means to ... the true enno-
blement of women, the full development of her unknown nature, and the
consequent redemption of the whole human race.*

Strictly speaking, Elizabeth Blackwell was not the first woman to practice medicine. Women have always practiced medicine either openly or
secretly. Before Elizabeth Blackwell, Harriot Kesia Hunt (1805–1875) practiced medicine for about 20 years in Massachusetts before she was allowed to
attend lectures at the Harvard Medical School in 1850. Hunt received an honorary M.D. from Women's Medical College of Pennsylvania in 1853. However, the medical schools did not open for women because of her. By modern
western educational and credentialing standards, Elizabeth Blackwell was the
first woman in the world to earn an M.D. degree from an accredited medical
school, satisfying the standard requirements of a full course of study. During her career, she faced many difficulties in practicing medicine on an equal
footing with men. Her continued fight against the odds enabled her to tremendously promote education of women and to open the doors of medical schools
to women.

Elizabeth Blackwell was born on February 3, 1821, in Counterslip, Bris-
tol, Gloucestershire, England, to Samuel Blackwell and Hannah Lane Blackwell. Mr. and Mrs. Blackwell had eleven children, and three of them died in
infancy. Mr. Samuel Blackwell was a sugar refiner who believed strongly that
all humans were created equal. With his wife's support, he actively participated in social reforms to enhance the social equality of all walks of life. As
a result, the Blackwell children were nurtured by open and liberal minds.
Several became pioneers and leaders in social reforms including promoting
women's professional status in many walks of society. For example, among

Elizabeth's sisters, Anna became a newspaper correspondent; Emily, a physician, helped Elizabeth greatly in promoting women's education; and Ellen became an author and artist. Elizabeth had two brothers who were also strong reformers. One of them, Samuel, was married to Antoinette Brown (1825–1921), who became the first ordained woman minister in America. Another brother, Henry, was married to Lucy Stone, who became an abolitionist and women's rights advocate. Elizabeth grew up in an enlightened family and was destined to have an unusual career, which would make a difference in society.

Samuel Blackwell tried to give the best education to his children. Both the boys and the girls were taught by private tutors. Unfortunately, Samuel didn't have a prosperous life. His sugar refinery was destroyed by fire in 1832 when Elizabeth was 11 years old. Following this disaster, the whole family moved to the United States in search of a better life. They spent the first six years in New York City and Jersey City. Even though they had financial difficulties, Elizabeth still received a good education. Daily, she was able to attend a very good school in New York.

The Blackwell family was totally against slavery, and they were involved in the anti-slavery movement. Their home often served as a haven for fugitives. The well known crusader William Lloyd Garrison (1805–1879) was a frequent visitor to their home.

In 1838 the Blackwell family moved to Cincinnati, Ohio, but unfortunately, Samuel Blackwell died shortly thereafter. Resourcefully, Mrs. Hannah Blackwell and her children opened a boarding school and tutored private pupils for a living. After struggling for four years, Elizabeth Blackwell took a teaching position at a girls' school in western Kentucky.

When Elizabeth reached marriage age, she felt little attraction to men and discouraged a tenacious suitor. She was more concerned with social inequalities, and she believed that men and women were entitled to equal opportunities in education. Although she enjoyed teaching, the desire of achieving a higher goal was in her mind. As expressed in her diary, she felt "the want of a more engrossing pursuit."

The idea of becoming a physician came to her mind while she was visiting a family friend, Mary Donaldson, who had cancer. Donaldson convinced her that female doctors would be better able to attend to the medical needs of women. Donaldson said, "If I would have been treated by a lady doctor, my worst sufferings would have been spared me." She encouraged Elizabeth to become a doctor by saying, "You have health, leisure, and a cultivated intelligence. Why don't you devote these qualities to the service of suffering women? Why don't you study medicine?"

The idea of earning a medical doctor's degree grew strong in Elizabeth's mind. She began to prepare herself to study medicine by reading medical texts diligently. She obtained a teaching post in Asheville, North Carolina, where she studied medicine privately with Dr. John Dickson. The year after, she taught music in Charleston, South Carolina, while continuing her studies with John's brother, Dr. Samuel Dickson. By 1847, she began to write letters to several prominent doctors asking them if they could help her to get into a medical school. One of the doctors to whom Blackwell wrote was Dr. Joseph Warrington, a well-respected physician in Philadelphia, Pennsylvania. Dr. Warrington replied to Blackwell's request. In the letter, he wrote that if the desire for her to become a medical doctor was a divine call, it would sooner or later be accomplished. Blackwell found Dr. Warrington's letter encouraging. She thought that she had a better chance of getting into a medical school if she moved to Philadelphia, where Dr. Warrington practiced. In May of 1847 she traveled to Philadelphia and introduced herself to Dr. Warrington, who was impressed by her earnestness and determination. He offered her the use of his private medical library and invited her to attend his medical lectures. They became good friends, and Dr. Warrington asked her to accompany him on some of his house calls. He also wrote letters of recommendation for her when she applied to medical schools.

Trying to get into medical school was not easy for women. In the early summer of 1847 Blackwell sent applications to many medical schools. She had already been turned down by schools in Philadelphia and New York, as well as Harvard, Yale, and Bowdoin. She was finally accepted by the Geneva Medical College (the precursor of the Syracuse Health Science Center College of Medicine) in west central New York State. Her admission to this school was an interesting episode.

The dean of the Geneva Medical College at the time was Dr. Charles Alfred Lee (1801–1872). He opposed the idea of accepting a female student, but he knew that Dr. Joseph Warrington was a well-respected physician. Dr. Lee did not want to displease Dr. Warrington. He thought that his students would not like to accept female students, so he placed the responsibility for rejecting Blackwell onto the student body by allowing them to vote on the matter. It was a surprise to the dean and the university faculty that students voted to accept her. According to Stephen Smith, a medical student at the time, the students did not know whether to take Dr. Lee seriously, and many thought that he was playing a practical joke. The students joined in the joke by voting yes unanimously. The astonished faculty, against their will but bound by their word of honor, had no choice but to accept her. Elizabeth seized the opportunity to go to medical school.

When she appeared on the campus on November 6, 1847, the students gave her a manly welcome; however, the doctors' wives and townspeople were unhappy. A few days after the semester started, she was informed by Professor James Webster that she would not be allowed to attend the classroom of dissecting because he thought it would be an embarrassment for a woman to be present when he covered the topic of the reproductive system. She protested and explained with good reasons why she should attend the class. Professor Webster took back his statement and confessed to the whole class that he had been justly rebuked. Following that incident, Professor Webster became her friend and supported her forthrightly. But that wasn't the situation of the entire community. Doctors' wives refused to speak to her. Many town women would draw their skirts aside as she passed them on her daily walks through town. Some stared at her as if she were an exotic species or regarded her as insane. Professor James Hadley, a registrar, promised her letters of recommendation but never sent the letters.

In 1848 she spent some time in a Philadelphia hospital doing clinical training. Her experience was a very negative one, as Elizabeth recalled in her autobiography. Although the medical head of the hospital was kind to her, the young resident physicians were not friendly. She was isolated and struggled with everything during her clinical study.

Despite being admitted as a practical joke and having to deal with an adverse environment, Blackwell graduated at the top of the class. On January 29 of 1849 she received her M.D. degree. When President Benjamin Hale handed her the diploma, she said, "Sir, by the help of the Most High, it shall be the effort of my life to shed honor on this diploma."

Blackwell's graduation from medical school produced a widespread effect in America. The public generally expressed a favorable opinion. Many women began to apply to medical schools and some of them were accepted. Medical schools seemed to begin opening doors for women.

However, this was not the case in the Geneva Medical College. Dr. Charles Lee gave the valedictory address at Blackwell's commencement. Although he praised the thoroughness and integrity of Dr. Blackwell's study of medicine, he said, "Such cases must ever be too few, to disturb the existing relations of society, or excite any other feeling on our part than admiration at the heroism displayed, and sympathy, for the sufferings voluntarily assumed." In other words, Lee and most of his colleagues would not like to see any other woman ever receive a degree in medicine. Geneva Medical College would no longer accept female medical students.

A vigorous debate about women physicians took place in the *Boston Medical and Surgical Journal* (now the *New England Journal of Medicine*). Dr.

Lee defended his position (speaking of himself in the third person), saying that he

> acknowledged the validity of the argument, so far as it is founded on the general physical disqualifications of the sex for the medical profession, and the incompatibility of its duties, with those probably belonging to the female portion of society, believes nevertheless, that instances occasionally happen, where females display such a combination of moral, physical, and intellectual qualifications for discharging creditably and skillfully the duties belonging to our calling, that it would seem equally unwise and unjust, to withhold from them those advantages and those honors, which are open to nearly all others, whether deserving of them or not. While he holds this opinion, he at the same time feels bound to say, that the inconveniences attending the admission of females to all the lectures in a medical school, are so great, that he will feel compelled on all future occasions, to oppose such a practice, although by so doing, he may be subjected to the charge of inconsistency.

We can see that even though Elizabeth Blackwell broke the ice for women to get equal education, there were still a lot of hindrances. Emily Blackwell, her sister, applying to get into the Geneva Medical College, was turned down. Instead, Emily went to the Western Reserve Medical College in Cleveland, Ohio, and got her M.D. degree there.

After graduation, Dr. Elizabeth Blackwell returned to Philadelphia for a few months and was naturalized as a United States citizen. Although her previous hospital grudgingly allowed her further study, her advancement as a physician was still much deterred. She was determined to become a surgeon and in 1849 decided to go to Europe to further her endeavor. She hoped to study with one of the leading French surgeons in a Parisian hospital but was denied access because of her gender. Instead, she enrolled in the state-run La Maternité, where she completed a midwifery course. The midwifery courses were very intensive and often involved extremely ill infants. In the summer of 1849, while attending to a child with gonorrhea, Dr. Blackwell inadvertently splashed some pus from the child's eyes onto her left eye. Dr. Blackwell contracted *ophthalmia neonatorum*, which led to the loss of vision in one eye. This accident put an end to any hopes of becoming a surgeon.

Dr. Blackwell could not accomplish anything or even gain recognition in Paris. In October of 1850 Dr. Blackwell left France for London where she studied at St. Bartholomew's Hospital under Sir James Paget. While in London, Dr. Blackwell became friends with Lord George Gordon Byron (1788–1824) and Barbara Leigh Smith, who were interested in promoting the education of women in England. Dr. Blackwell also established a lifelong friendship with Florence Nightingale (1820–1910), who was a heroine in the Crimean War (1854–1856). Through Nightingale's influence, she became interested in social causes, especially those regarding the political and educational status of women. Dr. Blackwell wholeheartedly agreed with Nightingale's viewpoint that sanitation was a crucial goal in medicine. However, Nightingale was only interested in promoting the status of nurses and establishing a modern nursing school, whereas Dr. Blackwell was more interested in promoting the opportunities for women to participate in all medical professional activities including being medical doctors. Dr. Blackwell's viewpoint on women's role in medicine was ahead of Nightingale's.

Dr. Blackwell had a strong attraction to her native land and intended to stay in London to practice medicine. However, she had neither capital nor support from friends to make it happen. In 1851 she was urged to go back to New York where she attempted to practice medicine. She was consistently blocked in achieving her goal. Fortunately, because of her social and professional connections, she was asked to give a series of lectures on hygiene to a group of highly influential ladies including some members of the Society of Friends, a Quaker organization. This opportunity gave her the first start in the practicalities of medical life. She also wrote and delivered a series of papers on the importance of good hygiene. Her series of lectures were published in 1852. The warm and permanent interest of her audiences gave her enormous encouragement, which lasted throughout her life.

Because no one would rent space for her practice, her career as a medical practitioner was not bright. In 1853, with the support of Lady Byron, Dr. Blackwell purchased a house in a run-down section of New York and opened a dispensary. This was a big adventure. She began to exert her influence with an increasing number of patients. She paid special attention to those who lacked options. In 1854 Dr. Blackwell adopted a seven-year-old Irish orphan, Katherine (Kitty) Barry, who remained her lifelong companion. In the same year, she was joined by Miss Marie Zakrzewska (1829–1902), a German immigrant who had been chief of midwifery at the Royal Hospital in Berlin. Marie Zakrzewska later obtained her M.D. degree from Case Western Reserve University in Cleveland, Ohio. In 1856 Emily Blackwell, Elizabeth's sister, by that time also a medical doctor, joined in her effort.

On May 12, 1857, the one-room dispensary received its first patients as the New York Infirmary for Women and Children. The Infirmary had a shaky start, but many reformers as far away as France and Boston had contributed funds toward its survival. The infirmary served as a training ground for newly graduated female doctors.

In 1858 Blackwell went to London again to further the cause of women's education in England. She lectured extensively and became the first woman to have her name entered in the British Medical Register. During this period of time, she convinced Elizabeth Garrett Anderson (1836–1917) to study medicine. Anderson later became a pioneer of English female doctors and contributed significantly to women's education in England.

Dr. Blackwell returned to America and her infirmary developed rapidly. Her plan to implement a medical college and nursing school for women into the infirmary was delayed because of the Civil War.

During the Civil War, with the guidance and support of Nightingale, Elizabeth and Emily Blackwell set up the Women's Central Association of Relief to train nurses in New York. Soon this association became the United States Sanitary Aid Commission officially appointed by President Abraham Lincoln (1809–1865). As this organization expanded, the Blackwells withdrew from further participation. They were more interested in women's medical education.

In September of 1862, the Emancipation Proclamation was issued and violent riots broke out in New York City in July of 1863. Some white infirmary patients demanded that the Blackwells discharge several black expectant mothers who had escaped from the South. The Blackwells stood firm on their purposes and refused to comply.

In 1868 the new Women's Medical College of the New York Infirmary was finally established. Dr. Blackwell served as a professor of hygiene, and her sister Emily's excellent managerial skills insured success. This was the first school devoted entirely to the medical education of women. It later became one of the first medical schools in America to mandate four years of study. It is also worth mentioning that the first black woman to become a medical doctor, Rebecca Cole (1846–1922), was one of the first graduates of the Women's Medical College. In 1869 Dr. Blackwell returned to England and left Emily to run the hospital and the college. Emily Blackwell served as dean of the college for thirty years.

The Blackwells established the Women's Medical College out of necessity, but they believed strongly that medical education should be co-educational. In 1898 when the new Cornell University Medical College was ready to accept women on equal terms, Emily Blackwell arranged to transfer students of Women's Medical College to Cornell, and thus closed the Women's Medical College. In this period, many other women's medical colleges also closed. As a consequence of these closings, there was a remarkable decline in the number of available positions for women physicians.

Dr. Blackwell began practicing medicine in England in 1869 and helped establish the National Health Society in 1871. In 1875 she accepted a professorship of gynecology at the New Hospital (now called the Royal Free Hospital) of the London School of Medicine for women. She was the first woman to be placed on the British Medical Register and taught at England's first college of medicine for women.

Because her health was deteriorating, Dr. Blackwell was forced to spend some time in Italy recuperating. As she grew older, she spent more and more time in a retreat in the highlands of Scotland. In 1907 she had a serious fall from which she never recovered. She died on May 31, 1910, in Hastings, England, and was buried in Kilmun, Scotland, a place that she and daughter Kitty enjoyed visiting in later life.

Neither Elizabeth Blackwell nor her sister Emily ever married. Emily adopted a daughter by the name of Anne. Emily and her colleague Elizabeth Cushier set up housekeeping together and established a companionable relationship. Emily died of enterocolitis on September 7, 1910, in her summer home at York Cliffs, Maine.

Elizabeth Blackwell was a prolific writer. Her doctoral dissertation was on the louse-borne typhus and was published in 1849 in the *Buffalo Medical Journal*. Many of her other writings are listed below. Her writings were influenced by the issues of her day.

For most of her life, Dr. Blackwell endeavored to make medicine an acceptable profession for women. However, she believed that the duty of women in the medical profession was not to imitate male medical practitioners but to define what was morally right and wrong in medicine for women. She was strongly convinced that the entrance of women into medicine made the profession in general more moral, that is, more responsive to a wide variety of human needs than men alone recognized. To Elizabeth and Emily Blackwell, practicing medicine was not their only goal in life but was a tool for fighting social injustices. Elizabeth assumed the responsibility of combating the inequities against women in the Victorian time.

* * *

Today, when women enjoy the possibility of equal participation in all professions, we should not forget Dr. Elizabeth Blackwell as a pioneer in making medicine an acceptable profession for women. Her contribution was not limited to the practice of medicine; she improved humanity in general by helping to tear down the walls separating sexes and races. Since she emphasized the importance of personal hygiene and crusaded for moral reforms in the medical profession, she contributed substantially to the progress of public health.

Further Reading

Baker, R. 1944. *The First Woman Doctor: The Story of Elizabeth Blackwell, M.D.* New York: Messner.

Fuller, W. 2003. Woman attends medical school. *Old News* (May and June). http://campus.hws.edu/his/blackwell/biography.html

Luft, E.V.D. Celebrating 150 years of women in medicine: the legacy of Elizabeth Blackwell. *Alumni Journal, the Publication of the Syracuse Medical Alumni Association.*

Morantz-Sanchez, R. 1992. Feminist theory and historical practice: rereading Elizabeth Blackwell. *History and Theory* **31**: 51–69.

_____. 1985. *Sympathy and Science: Women Physicians in American Medicine.* New York: Oxford University Press.

Sanes, S. 1944. Elizabeth Blackwell: her first medical publication. *Bulletins of the History of Medicine* **16**: 83–88.

Selected Publications of Elizabeth Blackwell

1. *Medicine and Morality* (1850)
2. *The Laws of Life with Special Reference to the Physical Education of Girls* (1852)
3. *An Appeal in Behalf of the Medical Education of Women* (published anonymously, 1856)
4. *Address on the Medical Education of Women* (1856)
5. *Medicine as a Profession for Women* (coauthored with Emily, 1860)
6. *Address on the Medical Education for Women* (co-authored with Emily, 1864)
7. *How to Keep a Household in Health* (1871)
8. *The Religion of Health* (1878)
9. *Counsel to Parents on the Moral Education of Their Children* (1878, second edition published in 1879 as the *Moral Education of the Young in Relation to Sex, Under Medical and Social Aspect*)
10. *Christian Socialism* (1882)
11. *Rescue Work in Relation to Prostitution and Disease* (1882)
12. *Wrong and Right Methods of Dealing with Social Evil, as Shown by English Parliamentary Evidence* (1883)
13. *The Human Element in Sex* (1884)
14. *On the Decay of Municipal Representative Government* (1885)
15. *A Medical Address on the Benevolence of Malthus, Contrasted with the Corruptions of Neo-Malthusianism* (1888)
16. *The Influence of Women in the Profession of Medicine* (1889)
17. *Why Hygienic Congresses Fail* (1892)
18. *Pioneer Work in Opening the Medical Profession to Women* (1895)
19. *Scientific Method in Biology* (1898)
20. *Essays on Medical Sociology* (1899)

4

LYDIA FOLGER FOWLER
(1822–1879)

First American Woman to Receive a Medical Degree

Lydia Folger Fowler was the first American woman to receive a medical degree and the first to hold a professorship in a legally authorized school of medicine in the United States. Lydia was born before the development of modern medicine and the birth of microbiology. Her way of practicing medicine was unique. However, she made a significant contribution to the field of public health as well as to socioeconomics and was also a role model for the promotion of women's medical education. Her life experience, therefore, is worth studying.

Lydia Folger was born in Nantucket, Massachusetts, on May 5, 1822. She was a daughter of Gideon and Eunice Macy Folger. Gideon Folger (1780–1863) was a direct descendant of John Folger, who immigrated to the United States from England in 1635.

The story of the Folger family is an important part of the early American immigration history. The Folgers were American frontiersmen. They contributed greatly to the building of this nation. They had vision, intelligence, industry, integrity, and tenacity that permitted them to face the challenge of limited opportunities. Some of the Folger family members were well known. These included Benjamin Franklin (1706–1790), statesman, writer, and inventor; Lucretia Mott, the celebrated Quaker preacher, abolitionist, and suffragist; and Maria Mitchell (1818–1889), the eminent astronomer.

There is little known of the childhood of Lydia. But we know that she had a strong thirst for knowledge, which was a common trait in her family. She attended Wheaton Seminary in Norton, Massachusetts, from 1838 to 1839 and taught there from 1842 to 1844. In 1844 Lydia married Lorenzo Niles Fowler, who along with his brother Orson Squire Fowler was a leading exponent of phrenology in the United States.

Phrenology was a popular nineteenth century practice of determining a person's mental strengths, abilities, and personality traits from the shape of the skull. Exercise of specific parts of the brain or even manipulation of the skull could allegedly change or develop its faculties. Phrenology gained popularity among upper class intellectuals and scientists in Britain in the 1820s. As theories of phrenology spread to the U.S. in the 1830s, they merged with the reform-oriented and commercializing culture of America and moved from the realm of scholarly research into a more practical and popular science that focused on self-improvement. Lorenzo and Orson Squire Fowler promoted phrenology as a self-improvement practice along with other popular forms of moral and health reform such as vegetarianism, temperance, mesmerism, and hydropathy (water cure).

Lydia Fowler became identified with the Fowler brothers and worked with them in a team. She delivered lectures on anatomy, physiology, and hygiene as well as phrenology to groups of women. She wrote elementary textbooks on these subjects, which are still found in our libraries. These publications include *Familiar Lessons on Physiology* (1847), *Familiar Lessons on Phrenology* (1847), and *Familiar Lessons in Astronomy* (1848).

Is phrenology a true science? This question must have been disturbing for Lydia Fowler. She wanted to study medicine. Her path to medical school was not an easy one. It was, however, made smoother by the women's rights movement that occurred at that time. In reaction to the first women's rights convention, a group of medical men of eclectic persuasion at Rochester and another at Syracuse — not far from the Geneva Medical College at Seneca Falls, where the first female medical student, Elizabeth Blackwell, attended — organized the Central Medical College of New York at Syracuse, with the announced policy of coeducation. This was the first chartered medical school in the modern world to make coeducation a policy. It was opened on November 5, 1849. Lydia Fowler was one of the eight women students among the total 92 students for its first class.

During the second term, the college moved to Rochester, New York, and Lydia Fowler served as principal of the female department. In 1850 she graduated to become the second woman in the world, after the Englishwoman Elizabeth Blackwell, to receive a medical degree in the United States.

In 1851 Fowler was appointed professor of midwifery and diseases of women and children at the college, the first woman professor in an American college. However, the school was closed in 1852 because of financial reasons. From 1852 to 1860, Fowler practiced medicine in New York City. She gave lectures frequently to women on hygiene and physiology and championed further opening of the medical profession to women. She was also interested in women's rights and temperance movements. During 1860 and 1861, she studied medicine in Paris and London. However, the law in England restricted physicians with foreign diplomas to register in Great Britain unless they had been in practice prior to October 1858. Because Fowler did not spend her time and energy in the personal practice of medicine, she became the honorary secretary of a woman's temperance society and a district visitor of a London church. She also became familiar with social conditions of the day, which increased her power as a writer and lecturer on health and temperance. In 1862 she returned to the United States and became an instructor in clinical midwifery at the New York Hygeio-Therapeutic College conducted by Russell T. Trall (1812–1877). She taught obstetrics and delivered health lectures to large audiences of women. She also had a private practice in medicine and reached a high place in the professional world. It seemed that she and her husband had a bright future in New York City. But the lecture opportunities in Great Britain were so attractive that she and her husband and their daughter moved to London permanently in 1863.

Dr. Fowler was happy to be in London because Great Britain was a new environment to her. The life in London presented an excitement and a new challenge to which she responded in full. She was a contemporary of Charles Dickens (1812–1870) and was lecturing in England, Ireland, Scotland, and Wales while Dickens was lecturing in the United States. It was estimated that about 200,000 women in English-speaking countries attended her lectures.

Most importantly, Dr. Fowler lectured to large groups of women on medical subjects of vital importance to them and their families. Those subjects were in the field of preventive medicine, which is the foundation of modern medicine.

In addition to delivering lectures and publishing pamphlets, she wrote stories to promote her objectives. In spite of her time-consuming duties, she found time for literary expression. She published a temperance novel called *Nora: The Lost and Redeemed* in 1863, in which one of the major characters was a medical student. In 1865 she published *The Pet of the Household and How to Save It,* which was a collection of lectures on child care. In 1870 she also published *Woman and Her Destiny* and *Heart Melodies,* which was a collection of poems written during various periods of her life.

Dr. Lydia Fowler also produced good students. Dr. Sarah Adamson Dolley (1829–1909), who practiced medicine for 50 years at Rochester, New York, and Dr. Myra King Merrick (1825–1899), co-founder of the Homeopathic Hospital and Medical College for Women in Cleveland, Ohio, were her students.

Dr. Fowler was dedicated to her work and had a tight schedule that consumed her life. She died of pneumonia on January 26, 1879, at the age of 57.

Dr. Lydia Fowler had a sympathetic understanding of human nature.

Her personality as well as her knowledge of medicine attracted favorable reaction from her audience and undoubtedly helped her career. She was also a great asset to her husband and brother-in-law.

*   *   *

Dr. Fowler was born and raised before modern medicine and the birth of microbiology, and her education was limited by today's standards. She began her work in the world during a period of erratic "-isms," "-ologies," "-pathies," and medical and social vagaries, representing a widespread dissatisfaction with things as they were. The medical profession was, for example, divided on the question of therapeutics. In addition to regular practitioners to whom treatment was largely empirical and all too often "heroic," and to whom "laudable pus" was surgical benediction, there were homeopaths, eclectics, hydropaths, and physiopaths. There were dissident systems of medicine. All along the line, there was plenty of room for reform, and the leading reformers were actuated by a desire to improve the practice of medicine.

Despite the medical confusion, Dr. Fowler made a great contribution in the field of preventive medicine, which is of vital importance for human health. She contributed significant articles to medical journals: "Medical Progression" was published in the *Eclectic Medical and Surgical Journal*, and "Female Education" as well as "Suggestions to Female Medical Students" appeared in the *Journal of Medical Reforms* published by the Metropolitan Medical College. Her service as a physician, as well as her contribution as a medico-social writer and lecturer, was enormous in her time.

Further Reading

Lovejoy, Esther Pohl. 1957. The first American woman doctor. In *Woman Doctors of the World*. New York: Macmillan. 8–21.

Physiognomy and phrenology. http://www.newcastle.edu/au/discipline/fine-art/theory/race/phrenol.htm

Women in American History, s.v. Fowler, Lydia Folger. 1999. Encyclopaedia Britannica online. http://search.eb.com/women/articles/Fowler_Lydia_Folger.html

5

MARIE ELIZABETH ZAKRZEWSKA
(1829–1902)

Pioneer German-Born Physician

The fact that a woman of no extraordinary powers can make her way, by the simple determination that whatever she can do she will do, must inspire those who are fitted to do much, yet who do nothing because they are not accustomed to determine and decide for themselves.

I am not speaking of fame, nor do I think that my name, difficult though it be, will be remembered. Yet the idea for which I have worked, the seeds which I have tried to sow here and there, must live, spread, and bear fruit.

Dr. Marie Elizabeth Zakrzewska was a pioneer woman physician. She not only served as an obstetrician, gynecologist, and general practitioner, but she also trained several generations of women doctors in hospitals. She helped found the New York Infirmary for Women and Children (now called Beth Israel Medical Center) and, in Boston, the New England Hospital for Women and Children (now the Dimock Community Health Center).

Marie was born on October 6, 1829, in Berlin, Germany. Her father was Ludwig Martin Zakrzewski, who was born into the family of a Polish landowner. Mr. Zakrzewski was a descendant of the aristocratic Zakrzewski family. Mr. Zakrzewski had served in the Prussian army but had been discharged with a pension because of his very liberal views. Her mother was Caroline Fredericka Wilhelmina Urban, who counted among her immediate ancestors gypsies of the Lombardi tribe and whose mother had been a veterinary surgeon. Marie was the oldest of five sisters and one brother. The family lived in poverty in Berlin, supported only by Mr. Zakrzewski's pension.

After six years of schooling, she left the school and, like many other German girls, did housework, but she spent most of her spare time reading medical related books. In order to help support the growing family, Marie's mother entered the school for midwives at the Charité Hospital in Berlin. Marie accompanied her mother and stayed at the hospital for several months. Since she had access to a lot of medical literature, she developed a profound interest in medicine. She assisted her mother in learning midwife techniques and applied for admission to the midwifery program at the age of 18. Unfortunately, she was rejected due to her young age. She was persistent in her interest in medicine and continued to assist her mother in her studies. Her talent attracted the attention of Dr. Joseph Hermann Schmidt (1804–1852), head of the school. Two years later, Dr. Schmidt secured a position for Marie and took her as his private student. One year later, Dr. Schmidt made her his teaching assistant. Marie graduated in 1851 and in May of 1852, a few hours before he died, Dr. Schmidt appointed her as chief midwife and instructor in the hospital's school for midwives. Although Marie was a good teacher and midwife, her promotion caused a lot of jealousy and, lacking the support of her mentor, she resigned her position after only six months. A year later, Marie emigrated with a younger sister to the United States, expecting to find in America greater freedom for women to practice medicine.

Marie and her sister arrived in New York in May 1853 and were joined by a third sister in September the same year. She was offered a job as nurse by Dr. Reisig. The first year of life in the United States was meager, but they survived. They lived on the proceeds of a small knitting enterprise.

In May of 1854, Marie's life changed drastically. She was introduced to Dr. Elizabeth Blackwell (1821–1910), a pioneer woman medical doctor. Dr. Blackwell was impressed by her character and potential and took her on as an assistant. Dr. Blackwell persuaded her to learn English and recommended her for admission to Cleveland Medical College (Western Reserve College), from which her own sister Emily Blackwell (1826–1910) had recently graduated.

Marie Zakrzewska registered in October of 1854 and was welcomed by Mrs. Caroline M. Severance, who became a very good friend and also assisted her financially. At the medical school, although she was cordially received by Dean John J. Delamater, Marie did experience cold treatment from other students because of her gender. In March 1856 Marie received her M.D. degree and returned to New York to help Dr. Blackwell's endeavors.

In the beginning when Marie returned from Cleveland, the prejudice against women physicians in New York was so great that Marie could not even rent an office in which to practice. She finally set up an office in Dr. Blackwell's back parlor.

Dr. Zakrzewska together with Drs. Elizabeth and Emily Blackwell pursued plans to establish a hospital devoted to training women doctors who could not find such opportunities elsewhere. Dr. Zakrzewska devoted herself to seeking funds in Boston, Philadelphia, and New York. On May 12, 1857, their dreams were realized, and the New York Infirmary for Women and Children received its first patients. This was the first hospital staffed by women in the United States and perhaps in the world. For the first two years, Dr. Zakrzewska voluntarily served as resident physician and general manager. She took care of the growing numbers of patients in the dispensary. By 1859 the institution was financially sound.

In the same year, Dr. Zakrzewska accepted an offer from the New England Female Medical College of Boston to be professor of obstetrics and diseases of women and children. She eventually became resident physician of a new hospital. This college had been founded by Dr. Samuel Gregory (1813–1872) in 1848. Dr. Gregory considered "man-midwives" an affront to decency. He intended to train female practitioners who could give parturient women skilled attendance. However, the controversial Dr. Gregory knew next to nothing about medical education, and the faculty of his school was staffed with people of dubious backgrounds. It did not take long for Dr. Zakrzewska to notice the lack of general education of the faculty. She stressed the importance of good general education and the crucial role of science in medicine. Her views were far above Dr. Gregory's understanding and in addition, the school was in a poor financial situation under his management. Dr. Zakrzewska resigned her position in 1862, and Dr. Gregory closed his hospital and disbanded its board of trustees.

With the support and advice of a board of female managers and several of the college trustees, Dr. Zakrzewska built the clinical department of the New England Medical College into a small hospital and dispensary for women. She also founded a new institution, the New England Hospital for Women and Children, which opened on July 1, 1862. The institution's mission was to provide women with medical aid from competent physicians of their own sex and to provide educated women with an opportunity for practical study in medicine, as well as to train nurses. When Dr. Zakrzewska was no longer associated with Dr. Gregory, many medical leaders in Boston gave her consistent encouragement. There was considerable support from non-medical professional people, particularly those involved with women's rights movements in which Dr. Zakrzewska was interested. With Dr. Zakrzewska's efforts, the 10-bed hospital grew steadily and in 1864 had to be moved to a larger building. In 1872 the hospital was expanded considerably and moved to a nine-acre site in Roxbury. The old building was later named in honor of Dr. Zakrzewska and is still used as a hospital today.

In the beginning at the New England Hospital for Women and Children, Dr. Zakrzewska was a resident physician, but she soon handed the job over to Dr. Lucy Sewall. Dr. Zakrzewska then became attending physician until 1887. Afterward, she became an advisory physician. Strongly supported by the board of directors including Lucy Goddard, Edna D. Cheney (1824–1904), and Samuel E. Sewall (Dr. Lucy Sewall's father), Dr. Zakrzewska played a leading role in the development of this hospital.

Because of the strong discrimination against women physicians, Dr. Zakrzewska thought that the New England Hospital's most important program was to give women physicians the best possible training. The staff of the hospital were all women because no other hospitals admitted women physicians in those days. She stressed the importance of good training and dedication to the profession. She perceived that neither sentimental sympathy nor a desire for status was an adequate motive for women to enter the medical field. She valued those with talents to practice medicine and praised those women physicians who were truly interested in scientific investigations. At first, some women without degrees studied medicine at the hospitals, but after 1881, all resident students were required to have M.D. degrees. The hospital maintained high standards, and many very competent women doctors completed their training at the New England Hospital for Women and Children. Dr. Zakrzewska was an invaluable source of inspiration to women doctors of her time.

After 1887 as she continued working as an advisory physician in the hospital, Dr. Zakrzewska built an extensive private gynecological practice. She suffered for several years from arteriosclerosis and heart attacks. She retired in 1899. On May 12, 1902, she died of apoplexy in her home in Jamaica Plains, Massachusetts. Her ashes were interred at the Forest Hills Cemetery according to her will.

There were many tales about the childhood of Dr. Zakrzewska. For example, in her early childhood, when Marie played dolls with her younger sister Minna, she often told her that her dolls needed to be nursed and doctored, and she, as a young physician, cared for each one until it died. Her fantasy of playing with her dolls revealed her childhood imagination, which indicated her early awareness of disease and death.

When she was nine, she spent a year in an ophthalmic hospital as a companion to a blind cousin. She witnessed the inadequacies and injustices in hospital care, which gave her a desire to be a head nurse so that someday she could right the wrongs. At the age of ten, she contracted an eye infection herself and was placed under the care of a physician. Because of her curiosity, the physician encouraged her to accompany him on his hospital rounds. Even though she could not see, she could hear his questions and directions, and she was extremely impressed. When she regained her sight, the doctor gave her two books, one on the history of midwifery and the other on the history of surgery. She found both to be extremely interesting, and her ambition to become a doctor seemed to take root in her mind at that time.

Marie entered primary school at the age of five. Three years later she was enrolled in a school for young girls. She adopted her parents' advice to do the right thing and fear nobody. This caused her some trouble at school, as she noted in a memoir: "The teachers ... called me unruly because I would not obey arbitrary demands without being given some reason, and obstinate because I insisted on following my own will when I knew I was in the right." She never felt comfortable or accepted at school. She was often regarded as "ugly and naughty." She also thought of herself as "excessively ugly" with her "large nose overshadowing the undeveloped feature" of her face. She was ridiculed frequently. As she recalled, her aunt would say of unattractive people that they were "almost as ugly as Marie." In events requiring social graces, she was always quiet, shy, and awkward. She never made friends with girls or felt like approaching them. With boys, she said, "I was merry, frank, and self-possessed." With girls, she was isolated and unhappy. At the age of 12, she once had an attachment to one of her teachers, a man twenty years her senior. Unfortunately, this teacher died of tuberculosis. That was a blow to her emotionally. At home, she experienced the unequal treatment between boy and girl from her parents. Although she was a superior student who wanted to read in the evening, her father, despite being a free thinker, required her to do housework instead. Her brother, who disliked his studies, was compelled to do lessons. When Marie complained, she was told that because she was a girl, she "never could learn much." Luckily, despite her father's insistence that she should learn domestic skills, he wanted his daughter to be able to "earn" an independent and responsible likelihood rather than simply to marry. Her mother, a successful midwife, provided a role model for her. Undoubtedly, her childhood experiences and family background had greatly influenced her mental development and achievements.

Dr. Zakrzewska was an intelligent, persevering, and opinionated woman. She was sometimes quick-tempered about what needed to be done. She also had strong human sympathies and was devoted to the needs of the poor. In her early practice in Boston, she took charity cases seriously. In the beginning, she made her calls on foot, often to distant parts of the city, until 1885 when she acquired a horse and buggy. Despite her busy days at the hospital, she also had a private practice.

Although she was devoted to her hospital and medical practice, she was drawn into some social reforms such as the anti-slavery crusade. While still a student, she met the great American abolitionists Theodore Parker (1810–1860), William Lloyd Garrison (1805–1879), and Wendell Phillips (1811–1884), who later became her close friends; and she supported their anti-slavery movements. She also supported women's rights movements and became one of the first members of the New England Women's Club, where she gave a number of lectures on hygiene and related topics.

She was a close friend of Karl Heinzen (1809–1880), a radical German-American journalist, and his wife, who stayed at Dr. Zakrzewska's house in Roxbury for many years. She also shared her home with Julia A. Sprague, a devoted friend.

Dr. Zakrzewska was a free thinker and denied any belief in an afterlife. In her early years, she was anti–Christian. As C. Annette Buckel (1833–1912) said, she had "bitter contempt for the church and professed Christians" (*Woman's Journal*, Nov. 8, 1902). But she became more tolerant as she grew older.

* * *

Marie Zakrzewska was a brave woman. She excelled in her profession and opened the door for women who were interested in becoming physicians. During her life, gender discrimination was common for almost all professions. Against all odds, she bravely pursued a career that had not been ventured into by other women. Her strong determination and high standards won her the credit of a pioneer woman physician. Like many other women pioneers, she never married. She devoted her life to working for a better life for others.

Futher Reading

Abram, R. S. 1985. *Send Us a Lady Physician: Women Doctors in America 1835–1920*. New York: Norton.

Blake, J. B. 1971. Marie Elizabeth Zakrzewska. In *Notable American Women: The Modern Period: A Biographical Dictionary*. Edited by Barbara Sicherman and Carol H. Green with Ilene Kantrov and Harriette Walker. Cambridge MA: Belknap/Harvard University Press.

Drachman, Virginia G. 1984. *Hospital with a Heart: Woman Doctors and the Paradox of Separation at the New England Hospital 1862–1969*. Ithaca NY: Cornell University Press. 21–70.

Oakes, Elizabeth H., ed. 2002. *International Encyclopedia of Women Scientists*. New York: Facts on File. 396.

Victor, Agnes C., ed. 1972. *A Woman's Quest: The Life of Marie E. Zakrzewska, M.D.* New York: Arno.

Woman's Journal, November 8, 1902.

6

ELIZABETH GARRETT ANDERSON (1836–1917)

Pioneering British physician

Elizabeth Garrett Anderson was the first British woman to be certified as a physician. She was also the first woman to earn a medical doctor's degree from the University of Paris at Sorbonne. She served as both dean and president of the London School of Medicine for Women and founded the New Hospital for Women, which was renamed Elizabeth Garrett Anderson Hospital after her death. Interestingly, she was also the first female mayor in Britain.

Elizabeth Garrett was born June 9, 1836, in Whitechapel, London. She was the second of the twelve children of Newson and Louisa Dunnell Garrett. Mr. Newson Garrett ran a pawnbroker's shop in London. In 1841 the family moved to Aldeburgh, Suffolk, where Mr. Garrett purchased a corn and coal warehouse. His business was very successful, and he became rich by 1850. Mr. and Mrs. Garrett considered education important for their children. When Elizabeth was 13 years old, she and her sister Louise were sent to attend a boarding school called Academy for the Daughters of Gentlemen at Blackheath. She learned English and French well. Although she was an excellent student, science and mathematics were not part of the curriculum. Elizabeth studied only two years at the school. In those days, English girls were expected to stay at home and wait for marriage. Young Elizabeth was much disappointed at the situation because she felt strongly that she would like to have a meaningful life for herself even though she did not object to marrying the right person. She said, "I was a young woman living at home with nothing to do in what authors call 'comfortable circumstances.' But I was wicked enough not to be comfortable. I was full of energy and vigor and of the discontent that goes with unemployed activities. Everything seemed wrong to me."

In 1859 Elizabeth Garrett met Emily Davies (1830–1921) when she was staying with a family friend, Jane Crow, in London. Emily Davies was a young woman with strong opinions about women's rights. Emily Davies also introduced Elizabeth to other young women who had similar viewpoints about women's rights. Elizabeth was apparently influenced by them, and her desire of achieving a career of her own was strengthened.

In 1859 Elizabeth's perspective of life opened with hope when she met Dr. Elizabeth Blackwell (1821–1910), the pioneer American woman doctor. Through Dr. Blackwell's inspiration, Elizabeth Garrett began to pursue a career in medicine. Initially, she faced strong opposition from her family when she decided to do so. Nevertheless, her father soon became her strong supporter after learning of her commitment. However, there was no British university that would accept female medical students at that time. Instead, she began her medical training as a nurse at Middlesex Hospital in 1860. She became an excellent nursing student, and the resident physicians at Middlesex Hospital were impressed by her performance. Doctors allowed her to attend operations and follow on their rounds. However, she constantly received letters from relatives asking her to give up her plan to become a doctor. Elizabeth Garrett wrote about this pressure to Emily Davies on August 17, 1860. She said, "I have had a letter from my mother.... She speaks of my step being a source of life-long pain to her, that is a living death, etc. By the same post I had several letters from anxious relatives, telling me that it was my duty to come home and thus ease my mother's anxiety."

Her performance in the Middlesex Hospital was so excellent that male students were jealous of her. As described later by Louisa Garrett Anderson, daughter of Elizabeth Garrett, "Elizabeth obtained a certificate of honor in each class examination; she did so well indeed that the examiner in sending her the list added, 'May I entreat you to use every precaution in keeping this a secret from the students?' In June trouble arose, the visiting physician asked his class a question, none of the men could answer, and Elizabeth gave the right reply. The students were angry and petitioned for her dismissal, a counter-petition was sent to the committee but she was told she would be admitted to no more lectures although she might finish those for which she had paid fees."

In 1863 male doctors at Middlesex Hospital issued a statement on the subject of women doctors, saying, "The presence of a young female in the operating theatre is an outrage to our natural instinct and is calculated to destroy the respect and admiration with which the opposite sex is regarded."

Elizabeth Garrett remained undaunted. She diligently continued her study of medicine. In England, one must be listed in the Medical Register in order to practice medicine. The Medical Act passed in 1858 in England stated that a person must be licensed by the qualifying board of a British university in order to be listed on the Medical Register. This act would prevent Elizabeth Garrett from practicing medicine. However, the Licentiate of the Society of Apothecaries (L.S.A) would entitle its holder members to practice medicine, and the charter of the Society of Apothecaries had not specifically barred women from taking its licensing examination. In order to qualify for the membership of L.S.A., a candidate had to serve as a physician's apprentice for five years and attend a set number of courses. Elizabeth Garrett endeavored to fulfill these requirements and in 1865, she passed the examination. With the financial support of her father, she was able to establish a medical practice in London.

Before Elizabeth passed her examination, she applied to Aberdeen Hospital for medical training in July 1863. On July 29 she received the reply letter from the hospital saying, "I must decline to give you instruction in Anatomy.... I have a strong conviction that the entrance of ladies into dissecting-rooms and anatomical theatres is undesirable in every respect, and highly unbecoming.... It is not necessary for fair ladies to be brought into contact with such foul scenes.... Ladies would make bad doctors at the best, and they do so many things excellently that I for one should be sorry to see them trying to do this one."

The passing of the licensing examination of the L.S.A. by Elizabeth Garrett did not wake up the members of the society to the realization of the importance of gender equality in the medical profession. Instead, the Society of Apothecaries immediately enacted restrictions against women's taking the licensing examination.

Even though Elizabeth Garrett was free to practice medicine, she faced continuing prejudice in the medical field. Small wonder that Elizabeth was committed to women's rights. She joined with her feminist friends Emily Davies, Dorothea Beale (1831–1900), and Francis Mary Buss (1827–1894) to form a women's discussion group called the Kensington Society. In 1866 this group organized a petition asking Parliament to grant women the right to vote. Though rejected immediately, their petition did receive support from liberals such as John Stuart Mill (1806–1873) and Henry Fawcett (1833–1884). Mr. Fawcett became friendly with Elizabeth and even asked her to marry him. Elizabeth rejected his proposal because she believed it would damage her career. Mr. Fawcett later married Elizabeth's younger sister Millicent Garrett (1847–1929).

In 1866 Elizabeth entered the Medical Register and founded St. Mary's Dispensary for Women in London. Although Elizabeth Garrett became a physician, her L.S.A. degree was not generally regarded as esteemed as a medical degree. Elizabeth still desired the prestige conferred by the medical degree. She therefore pursued that desire after learning that the University of Paris at Sorbonne had begun to admit women. She reviewed her course work, further improved her French, and took several examinations. In 1870 she became the first women to earn a medical degree from the Sorbonne. In the same year, she was appointed a visiting physician to the East London Hospital. However, the British Medical Register did not recognize her M.D. degree.

During this period, Elizabeth Garrett was active in many women's issues and involved in a dispute with Josephine Butler (1828–1906), a well known women's rights supporter, concerning the Contagious Diseases Acts, which Dr. Elizabeth Garrett strongly supported. Dr. Garrett believed that the acts provided an important means of protecting women and children. However, Josephine Butler believed that the acts discriminated against women and felt that all feminists should support their abolition.

In 1870, the Education Act of England allowed women to vote and serve on school boards. Dr. Elizabeth Garrett obtained overwhelming support and won the top votes for the school board in London. The same year, Elizabeth Garrett applied for a position at the Shadwell Hospital for Children. Mr. James Skelton Anderson (1838–1907), a board member of the hospital and the financial adviser, was strongly opposed to her application. However, after interviewing her personally, he was so impressed that he fell in love with her. He eventually proposed to her, and they married in 1871. They had three children, Louisa, Margaret, and Alan. Margaret died of meningitis during childhood. Their marriage seemed to be a good one in the beginning. James Anderson supported Elizabeth's desire to continue as a doctor. But the couple became involved in a dispute when Mr. Anderson insisted on taking control of her earnings.

Dr. Elizabeth Garrett, now Dr. Elizabeth G. Anderson, continued her effort in medical practice. In 1872 she opened the New Hospital for Women in London. This hospital was staffed entirely by women. Dr. Elizabeth Blackwell (1821–1910), the woman who inspired her to become a medical doctor, was appointed professor of gynecology. In 1877 she and Dr. Sophia Jex-Blake (1840–1912) co-founded the London School of Medicine for Women. Dr. Jex-Blake expected to be put in charge of the school, but Dr. Anderson believed that her temperament made her not appropriate for the position. She arranged for Dr. Isabel Thorne to be appointed instead. In 1883 Dr. Anderson was elected dean of the school. During this time, Dr. Sophia Jex-Blake suffered the bitterness of betrayal and decided to establish the Edinburgh School of Medicine for Women in Scotland. In 1903 Elizabeth Anderson became president of the London School of Medicine for Women. She kept this job until her retirement.

In 1902, the Andersons retired to Aldeburgh, where Mr. James Anderson was elected mayor. Elizabeth Anderson continued her interest in politics.

James Anderson died in 1907 and Dr. Elizabeth Anderson completed his term. With her superb leadership, she was overwhelmingly elected mayor of Alde-burgh in 1908, the first woman mayor in the history of England. In the same year, she joined the Women's Social and Political Union (WSPU), which was a militant women's liberation organization campaigning for arson activities. She also joined with other members of the WSPU to storm the House of Com-mons the same year. She was lucky not to be arrested; many other members of the WSPU were not so lucky.

She left the WSPU in 1911 as she disagreed with their arson campaign. Her daughter Louisa Garrett Anderson (1873–1943) was also a member of WSPU. Unfortunately, Louisa was arrested and put in prison in 1912 for her militant activities. Louisa was also a medical doctor and left for France in 1914 to head a military hospital during World War I. Elizabeth G. Anderson died on December 17, 1917, at the age of 81.

Elizabeth had two sisters who achieved national celebrity. Millicent Gar-rett (1847–1929), who married Mr. Henry Fawcett, became the leader of the National Union of Women's Suffrage Societies, and Agnes Fawcett became a well known furniture designer.

* * *

Dr. Elizabeth Anderson's legacy was profound. The difficulty for a woman to become a medical doctor in her time was beyond description. She was not only a pioneer as a woman physician but also a great contributor to medical education as a whole and to women's education in particular. She was a good leader and a highly regarded administrator. Her creation of a med-ical school and hospital has tremendously enriched human welfare. She also served as a shining example to women trying to succeed in any field.

Further Reading

Education on the Internet & Teaching History Online. Http://www.spartacus.schoolnet. co.uk/WandersonE.htm

Oakes, Elizabeth H., ed. 2002. Anderson, Elizabeth Garrett (1836–1917). In *International En-cyclopedia of Women Scientists*. New York: Facts on File. 9–10.

7

ANNA W. WILLIAMS
(1863–1954)

Developer of Diphtheria Antitoxin and of a
Method for Quickly Diagnosing Rabies

Diphtheria was a deadly infectious disease without cure in the 1800s. In Europe, Emil von Behring (1854–1917) worked closely with Shibasaburo Kitasato (1856–1931) to develop a famous serum therapy and won the first Nobel Prize for Medicine or Physiology in 1901. Diphtheria was just as threatening in the United States as it was in Europe. Anna W. Williams was devoted to the study of this dreaded childhood disease, and her study led to the discovery of the *Corynebacterium diphtheriae* bacillus. Her work also led to the development of a rabies vaccine and an improved method of diagnosing rabies. She also helped build some of the most successful teams of bacteriologists, including many women working in the medical field in her time. Yet she was not rewarded for her accomplishments during her lifetime.

Anna Wessels Williams was born in Hackensack, New Jersey, on March 17, 1863. Her father was William Williams, and her mother was Jane Van Saun. Mr. Williams came from England and was a private school teacher. Jane Van Saun was from the Netherlands and supported the missionary activities of the First Dutch Reformed Church. They had six children including Anna. The financial burden was so strong that they could not afford for their children to attend private schools. Anna was schooled at home until she was twelve; then she entered the State Street Public School where Mr. Williams was a trustee. During this school period Anna first encountered the wondrous microscope, which opened her eyes to the microbial world. This experience might have been the beginning of her interest in microbial diseases. She then attended the New Jersey State Normal School and graduated in 1883. After graduation Anna taught school for the next two years.

In 1887 one of her sisters, Millie, almost died from the complications of delivering a stillborn child. This event was a big shock to Anna, and she decided to pursue a medical career because she vowed to prevent such incidents from happening again. In the same year, she attended the Women's

College of the New York Infirmary, which was created by Elizabeth Black-well (1821–1910). She studied obstetrics and gynecology under the direction of Dr. Blackwell and earned her medical degree in 1891. Also in 1891 she worked as an assistant to the Chair of Pathology and Hygiene at the New York Infirmary for Women and Children. From 1892 to 1893, Anna continued to pursue her medical education in Europe, studying at the universities of Vienna, Heidelberg, and Leipzig and interning at the Royal Frauen Klinik of Leopold in Dresden.

In 1894 Dr. Williams became an assistant bacteriologist in the newly established New York City Department of Health, the nation's first city-operated diagnostic laboratory under the directorship of Dr. William Hallock Park (1863–1939). At this time diphtheria was a leading cause of death among children. There was no effective treatment, and the death rate was on the increase. Williams and Park together conducted research on diphtheria with an aim to search for an antitoxin. Some time in 1894 while Park was on vacation, Williams independently isolated a disease-producing strain of *Corynebacterium diphtheriae* from a mild case of tonsillar diphtheria. This bacillus became the stock strain from which the first effective diphtheria antitoxin was prepared and made available to patients who could not afford it. Soon this antitoxin was used for immunization throughout North America and Great Britain. The isolation of this strain known as Park-Williams #8 (more commonly called "Park 8" strain) was generally credited to Park, even though he was not involved in the initial discovery. In 1895 Williams was promoted to assistant bacteriologist.

Williams then turned her attention to the study of other common diseases such as strep throat (commonly caused by *Streptococcus pyogenes*), pneumonia (primarily caused by *Streptococcus pneumoniae*), and scarlet fever (caused by *Streptococcus pyogenes*) in search for antitoxins. She also conducted diagnostic studies related to trachoma (caused by *Chlamydia trachomatis)* and other chronic eye infections generally found among the city's underprivileged children.

In 1896 Williams traveled to the Pasteur Institute in Paris, where she hoped to develop an antitoxin for scarlet fever. She took her diphtheria bacillus to the institute and in return, the scientists there helped her with her research. She collaborated with Dr. Alexander Marmorek (1865–1923) in streptococcal investigations. Her attempt to find antitoxins for scarlet fever was not successful. However, she turned her attention to rabies and collaborated with Dr. Emile Duclaux (1840–1904). Her experiments with a rabies virus culture were so successful that when she returned to the United States in 1898, she had a rabies vaccine with her, and it was mass-produced immediately.

Beginning in 1902 Dr. Williams collaborated with Dr. Alice G. Mann to search for ways to improve the means for diagnosing rabies and streptococcal diseases. She discovered a brain cell aberration specific to rabid animals. She improved the method of rabies diagnosis based on this discovery. Her method was far better than the existing method. About the same time, an Italian pathologist, Adelchi Negri (1876–1912), also independently worked on rabies and published the same discovery in 1904; hence, the name Negri body was used for these aberrant cells. Later in 1905 Williams announced her discovery of a method of staining the brain cells that allowed the near-instant diagnosis of rabies. Before the publication of her method, a diagnosis of rabies took about ten days. With her method diagnosis was made possible in less than half an hour. This method became a standard test for rabies for the next thirty years. The same year Williams was promoted to assistant director of the New York City Department of Health Laboratory. She continued to work for Dr. Park. Between 1902 to 1905 she was also a consultant to the New York Infirmary for Women and Children.

In recognition of the contribution of Dr. Williams, the American Public Health Association appointed Williams as chair of its newly-formed committee on the diagnosis of rabies in 1907. In 1914 Williams was elected president of the Women's Medical Society of New York. During World War I Williams served on the influenza commission and directed the training program at New York University for the War Department, which trained workers for medical laboratories at home and overseas. She also contributed to programs that detected meningococcal carriers in the military. In 1931 she was elected vice-chair of the laboratory section of the American Public Health Association. The next year she chaired the section, the first woman to hold this position.

Dr. Williams published many research papers over the course of her career. She was concerned with education because the knowledge about infectious diseases was not well disseminated. There was a lack of good textbooks at the time. With Dr. Park she co-authored the widely used *Pathogenic Microorganisms Including Bacteria and Protozoa: A Practical Manual for Students, Physicians and Health Officers*. This book became a classic text and sold 11 editions. In 1929 she and Park co-authored *Who's Who among the Microbes*. In 1932 she published her life's work, a monograph, *Streptococci in Relation to Man in Health and Disease*.

In addition to her groundbreaking research, she helped build successful teams of bacteriologists including many competent women who worked on various infectious diseases.

In 1934 Williams was forced to retire because New York City Mayor

Fiorella La Guardia (1882–1947) decreed mandatory retirement for all city employees over seventy years old. Since Dr. Williams' work was good and she was still in good health, her colleagues as well as other scientists urged La Guardia to allow Dr. Williams to continue her important research. However, the mayor refused to make an exception. Although she retired, she continued to work with Emily Dunning Barringer (1876–1961) toward better diagnosis and treatment of venereal diseases. She also collaborated with Sara Joseph Baker (1873–1945) in the Division of Child Hygiene to study eye infections affecting the poorest children in New York City.

She left New York City to live in Woodcliff Lake, New Jersey, and subsequently moved to Westwood, New Jersey, where she lived with her sister, Amelia Wilson. Williams died from heart failure on November 20, 1954, at the age of 91.

*   *   *

Despite the fact that Williams made great contributions, she didn't receive any significant awards or recognitions. Her isolating the disease-causing strain of *Corynebacterium diphtheriae* should be completely credited to her, yet the credit went totally to Dr. Park. Her method of rapid diagnosis of rabies was used for over thirty years; now it is hardly mentioned in any textbooks. She was never promoted beyond the position of the assistant director of the laboratory. If a male scientist had made the discoveries that she did, he would have received numerous honors and awards, or even a Nobel Prize. Gender discrimination is certainly one of the major factors of her mistreatment. Nevertheless, Dr. Williams was generous and broad-minded and had never been bothered by the unfair treatment toward her. She said that she was glad to have her name associated with Dr. Park's. Undoubtedly, she had a valuable and productive life. Because of her, we all live better.

Further Reading

Cook, Jane Stewart. 1995. Anna W. Williams. In *Notable Twentieth-Century Scientists*. Vol. 1. Edited by Emily J. McMurray et al. Detroit: Gale Research. 2211–2212.

Oakes, Elizabeth H., ed. 2002. *International Encyclopedia of Woman Scientists*. New York: Facts on File. 379–380.

8

MADAME MARIE
SKLODOWSKA CURIE
(1867–1934)

Discoverer of Medically Important Radium

I am one of those who think that science has great beauty. A scholar in his laboratory is not just a technician; he is also a child face to face with natural phenomena that impress him like a fairy tale.

A nation that does not invest in research is a nation on the decline.—Marie Sklodowska Curie (1867–1934)

Madame Curie was a renowned physicist and radiochemist. Her discovery of radioactive elements revolutionized the fundamental understanding of physics and chemistry. Her work also affected significantly the progress of medicine. Our regard for her as a woman pioneer in medical research is very appropriate. Madame Curie was the first woman professor in France. She was the only woman who won two Nobel prizes for science. Her life story is worthy to be studied.

Madame Curie was born in Warsaw, Poland, in 1867. Her original name was Marya Sklodowska. She changed her first name to its French form, Marie, when she was a student in France. Both her father, Vladislav, and her mother, Bronislawa, were teachers. Vladislav taught high school physics and mathematics. Bronislawa was a full-time director of a private school for girls. Marie was the last of their five children. Bronislawa had tuberculosis and quit her job after the birth of Marie. Because of her health problem, Bronislawa never kissed her youngest child in order to prevent the spreading of the disease. This lack of cuddling had a great influence on Marie's later mental development.

Marie's childhood was generally unhappy. Russia and Germany had divided Poland between them and were trying to destroy every vestige of Polish nationalism and culture. In Tsarist Poland, Marie learned early that expressing her emotions could be dangerous. The Poles lived a life without privacy that required silence and self-control. For this reason, Marie grew up hating loud voices, commotion, theatrics, and any display of emotion. However, the Sklodowskis were a passionate family of strong convictions. Bronislawa was an extremely devout Roman Catholic. The whole family was intensely patriotic and believed strongly in education. Madame Curie recalled, "My father and mother worshipped their professions in the highest degree." Marie learned to read before she was four years old.

When Marie was 11, her oldest sister, Sofia, died of typhus and her mother of tuberculosis. Because of her mother's health problem and aloof behavior toward her children, Marie idolized her mother. When her mother died, Marie fell into deep depression. She concluded that God did not exist and became an atheist.

During her school years, Marie experienced political intimidation and oppression because the Russians ran Polish schools like police states. Polish teachers were fired and students punished for speaking their own languages. Marie's father moved from school to school and apartment to apartment, each smaller than the last. They became so poor that her father had to take in student boarders for tutoring. The apartment became so crowded that Marie slept on a sofa in the dining room and got up early each morning to clear the room for the boarders' breakfast.

Despite all this hardship, Marie was the brightest student in her class. One of the unhappy things that she had to do was to cheat the Russian inspector. Whenever the government inspector arrived, Marie was chosen to be responsible for fooling the government inspector into thinking that her school taught Russian culture in Russian instead of Polish culture in Polish. Although Marie performed perfectly, she was so tense that, when the inspector left, she burst into tears. Because of this experience, she was nervous about public speaking for the rest of her life.

In secondary school, the situation was even worse. The Russian professors treated their Polish students like enemies. Madame Curie said, "The moral atmosphere was altogether unbearable." One of her brother's friends was hanged for political activities. Schools became centers of Polish nationalism and organized resistance. Education became a patriotic duty and moral imperative. An uprising against Russia occurred in 1863 but collapsed. A group of Warsaw intellectuals called Positivists campaigned for women's emancipation and education; science; toleration of Jews; abolition of class distinctions; reform of the Polish Roman Catholic Church; and education for the peasants. Women formed the backbone of the Positivist movement and founded the clandestine Flying University, where anyone could attend secret lectures in return for teaching one. Marie was strongly in favor of this movement. She said, "You cannot hope to build a better world without improving the individual." Her passionate commitment to hard work, learning, and science was inspired by the struggle for Poland's nationhood.

In 1882 at the age of fifteen, Marie graduated first in her class in every subject. In 1883 she collapsed; it was the first of several physical breakdowns that she suffered throughout her life. Her father arranged for her to take the year off, visiting relatives in the countryside and enjoying herself. She did enjoy the time. She said, "All I can say is that this will never happen again, never in my whole life, will I have such fun."

After a year of relaxed pleasure, she wanted to continue her education, but Russian government prohibited women from attending any university within its empire. Marie made a pact with her elder sister Bronya. Marie would work and support Bronya through medical school in Paris, and then Bronya would help pay Marie's way.

Not many jobs were available for girls at that time. Marie spent six years (1885–1891) as a governess — little more than a servant in a wealthy home. She lived with the Zorawski family sixty miles from Warsaw. She tutored two of the Zorawski children seven hours a day. She also taught local peasant children to read and write, an illegal activity for which she could have been severely punished. Mr. Zorawski permitted her to use the technical library in his sugar beet factory. She also used this opportunity to learn some chemistry from a factory chemist.

During this period of her life, she met Kazimierz, the eldest son of the Zorawskis and a student at the University of Warsaw. She was attracted to him and fell in love with him. However, the Zorawskis were appalled that their son and heir would consider marrying a mere governess; they forbade their engagement. Disappointed and trapped because Bronya needed money in Paris, Marie stayed in the Zorawskis' household for two and a half more years. She said, "Creatures who feel as keenly as I do — have to dissimulate it as much as possible — I would give half my life to be independent again, to have my own home."

In 1891 Marie finally gave up the dream to marry Kazimierz and left for Paris with forty rubles in her pocket. She enrolled in the University of Paris on November 5 of the same year. By then she had been out of school for eight years. Her French was inadequate, and she had studied less math and science than French high school graduates. She rented a sixth-floor garret room and lived on bread with occasional eggs, fruit, and cups of hot chocolate. She was very poor, but she regarded this as a heroic period because she had space of her own, privacy, independence, and as much time as she wanted to study. She said, "This life, painful from certain points of view, had, for all that, a real charm for me. It gave me a very precious sense of liberty and independence."

This heroic period lasted for two years, and in 1893 she earned the equivalent of a master's degree in physics and ranked top in her class. She was also awarded a Polish fellowship of six hundred rubles a year. In 1894 she obtained a similar degree in mathematics and ranked second in her class.

By a stroke of good fortune in 1894, Marie met Pierre Curie (1859–1906) at the home of a Polish physicist located in Paris. Pierre Curie was the laboratory director of the Municipal School of Industrial Physics and Chemistry in Paris. His research specialized in crystals and magnetic materials. When they first met, Marie was attracted to his auburn crewcut, limpid eyes, grave smile, and simple manners. His conversation about physics and social issues fascinated her. Pierre saw her as a Slavic beauty, much in vogue at the time, with curly blonde hair, gray eyes, wide cheekbones, and a broad forehead. In particular he saw her brilliance and passion for physics. They exchanged addresses the first day they met and had dinner together. Pierre gave Marie a new book by Emile Zola (1840–1902) that had just been banned by the Catholic Church. They quickly fell in love with each other. Marie still dreamed of returning to Poland to teach physics. However, Pierre persuaded her that she could do more and better research in France than in impoverished Poland. He said, "It is necessary to make a dream of life, and to make a dream a reality." They were married in 1895 without rings, blessings, or priests. Among their wedding presents were two bicycles, and, wearing a split skirt and a black straw hat, Marie took off with Pierre on the first of many bicycle tours.

Eventually, Pierre finished his doctoral dissertation on the relationships between temperature and the magnetic susceptibilities of paramagnetic substances, which is now known as Curie's law.

After marriage, Marie studied for a teaching certificate in order to qualify as a professor in girls' high schools. In August 1896 she passed the teacher's examination and obtained financial support from the metallurgical industry to study the magnetic properties of steel. In addition, she continued to work toward a doctorate.

Finding a research topic for a dissertation was not easy in physics. In 1896 radioactivity in uranium was discovered by Henri Becquerel (1852–1908), but few scientists paid great attention to this discovery. Becquerel's radiation occurs when the heavy, unstable nucleus of an atom breaks apart and ejects its excess energy as clusters of protons and neutrons (called alpha particles), as super fast electrons, or as gamma rays of pure energy. X-ray was discovered in 1895, originating in the clouds of electrons surrounding each atom. X-ray is much less powerful than the uranium radiation. Marie was interested in this new discovery and decided to work on Becquerel's radiation for her dissertation topic. Pierre was extremely helpful to her interest and secured a space at his college for her research.

Becquerel had demonstrated that radiation coming from the element uranium could blacken photographic plates, even those wrapped in heavy cardboard. He also showed that uranium makes the air around it conduct electricity. Marie recognized that as an ionization, which could be used to detect radioactivity in other substances. She examined whether any other known elements could also produce radioactivity. She used the piezoelectric quartz balance discovered by Pierre to measure the weak electrical charges. Through the close collaboration between Pierre and Marie, they discovered that another element, thorium, produces radioactivity as powerful as uranium. During the same time, she measured the strength of the electrical current produced by different uranium and thorium compounds. She also discovered that radioactivity does not depend on how atoms are arranged into molecules; instead, radioactivity originates within the atoms themselves.

Marie extended her research beyond uranium and thorium and their simple compounds to natural ores. She discovered that two uranium ores — pitchblende and chalcolite — were three and four times more radioactive than could be predicted from the amount of uranium or thorium they contained. She hypothesized the presence of an unknown highly radioactive element in the ore and coined the new word "radioactivity."

In April of 1898 Marie published her findings. About this time, Pierre dropped his crystal research and joined Marie's radioactivity project. Together they found the third radioactive element called polonium, which was named by her in honor of her native land. At the end of 1898 she discovered another more active element called radium. The discovery of radioactive polonium and radium was published in July and December of 1898, and she was awarded thirty-eight hundred francs by the French Academy of Sciences.

Marie's contribution was not only the discovery of new radioactive elements, but she also opened a new field of physics — radioactivity, which became the primary technique for exploring the interior of the atom. She and Pierre spent much time and effort isolating and purifying radium from ore. It was labor intensive. She said, "Sometimes I had to spend a whole day mixing a boiling mass with a heavy iron rod nearly as large as myself. I would be broken with fatigue at that day's end." Marie and Pierre worked together, sharing their physics and chemistry knowledge, but Marie was the driving force. She directed lab discussions and kept the operation going, while Pierre added scientific concepts.

The laboratory was in poor condition. The space was not adequate and there was no ventilation system for removing poisonous fumes. Also the roof leaked. Marie was sick with pneumonia or some other serious illness, often for several months at a time.

Despite the hard work and the poor laboratory conditions, Marie was very happy. She said, "It was in this miserable old shed that the best and happiest years of our life were spent, entirely consecrated to work." She was also extremely happy with Pierre. She said, "He was as much and much more than all I had dreamed at the time of our union. My admiration of his unusual qualities grew continually."

Marie and Pierre worked extremely hard to isolate radium from pitchblende. Marie also had to commute weekly to Sèvres to give lectures at a teachers' training college for women. By September 1902 they had isolated one-tenth gram of radium chloride from several tons of pitchblende. She also determined the atomic weight of radium at 226.

The discovery of radium opened a new field of physics. Before, physicists assumed that atoms were solid, indivisible, stable, and immutable. But radium proved that some powerful forces exist inside the atom. Ernest Rutherford (1871–1937) demonstrated that atoms of radioactive substances could change from one element to another. The definition of element faced challenge. Scientists began to recognize a new force of nature.

The honors and reputations of the Curies began to spread. Pierre Curie was invited to give a talk at the Royal Institution in London in June 1903. During his talk, Pierre began to have violent joint pain, and his legs and fingers began to tremble. As he demonstrated the properties of radium and radioactivity, he fumbled, spilling some of Marie's radium. The podium was contaminated with radioactivity that was not decontaminated until fifty years later.

Marie was so concentrated on her research that she didn't defend her dissertation titled "Researches on Radioactive Substances" until June 1903. That evening after the defense, the Curies celebrated with their friends, Paul Langevin (1872–1946), Jean Perrin (1870–1946) and his wife, and Ernest Rutherford. That evening, it was discovered that Pierre had serious rheumatism.

In the same year, the French Academy of Sciences nominated Henri Becquerel and Pierre Curie to be candidates to share the Nobel Prize for Physics for the work on radioactivity. Marie was not included. This caused the objection of one of the most powerful Swedish mathematicians on the nominating committee, Magnus Gosta Mittage-Leffler (1846–1927), who was a great supporter of women scientists. He wrote Pierre that he and he alone was being considered for the prize. Pierre cared little about prizes himself, but he wanted his wife to get credit for her work. So he wrote back to the committee, "If it is true that one is seriously thinking about me (for the prize), I very much wish to be considered together with Madame Curie with respect to our research on radioactive bodies." He also added with Gallic logic, "Don't you think that it would be more artistically satisfying if we were to be associated in this manner?" However, Marie Curie was not nominated for the 1903 prize. Nevertheless, she received two nominations the previous year, which was considered still valid. So the committee declared that Marie and Pierre Curie and Henri Becquerel were the Nobel Laureates for Physics in 1903. The Curies were too sick to collect their prize in December 1903. It was eighteen months later that Pierre was able to give the obligatory lecture and pick up their prize money.

The discovery of radium was enthralling to the public. It was regarded as a possible cure against cancer; and it was magical, changing from one element into another and producing a seemingly inexhaustible energy supply. By the end of 1903 Marie Curie was a household word. Reporters packed the Curies' front step, hoping for exclusive interviews. The Curies were overwhelmed. Pierre said in July 1905, "For a year now I have done no work, and I haven't had a moment to myself." "Obviously," he added, "I haven't found a way to protect us from frittering away our time, and yet I must. It's a matter of life and death intellectually."

However, Marie led a very active life, between her children, the School at Sèvres, and the laboratory. She still resented the inadequacy of their laboratory. She and Pierre had published thirty-six research papers between 1898 and 1904. Both of them turned down enticing offers from the University of Geneva in Switzerland. Nevertheless, in 1904 Pierre became a professor at the prestigious Sorbonne, a part of the University of Paris, which promised him a laboratory. Marie became a professor at the women teacher's college at Sèvres and was told she would become superintendent of Pierre's laboratory when it was built at Sorbonne. But the construction of the laboratory had not even begun in 1906. When Pierre was offered the Legion of Honor, he refused it, saying, "I do not in the least feel the need of a decoration, but I do feel the greatest need for a laboratory." On April 19, 1906, Pierre was hit by a horse drawn wagon when he crossed a busy street in the rain while trying to open his umbrella. His skull was crushed, and he died at the age of 48.

Marie Curie refused to receive a pension from the University of Paris because she did not want to be considered a dependent of Pierre. The University of Paris offered her a position as an assistant lecturer at ten thousand francs yearly starting in May 1906. It was her first university salary, and she was the first woman professor in France. On November 5, 1906, she gave her first lecture. As usual she was nervous when speaking in public. The newspaper editor wrote, "The magnificent forehead was noticed first. It was not merely a woman who stood before us, but a brain — a living thought."

Between 1903 and 1906, Marie faced a scientific challenge. Lord Kelvin (1824–1907) wrote to the editor of the *Times* and claimed that radium was not an element but a compound of lead and helium. Lord Kelvin was well known. His doubts regarding the element radium were devastating to Curie. She could not prove him wrong because she isolated radium chloride in 1902, and she had not produced pure radium. She then began arduously to purify the radium. With enormous persistence and determination for four years, she finally produced a few grams of pure radium and proved that radium is indeed an element.

In 1908 she became a full professor of general physics. In November 1911 Madame Curie was nominated by Svante Arrhenius for a Nobel Prize in Chemistry. It is believed that the Nobel Committee had paved the way for her in 1903 when she shared the Nobel Prize with Antoine H. Becquerel and Pierre Curie. The Nobel Committee excluded the discovery of radium as a part of the Nobel Prize in 1903. The Nobel Prize in 1911 was offered for the discovery of radium, which was done exclusively by Marie Curie. She received the award without Pierre this time.

In 1911 Marie sought election to the prestigious French Academy of Sciences. As a member of the Academy, she would be able to present research at the Academy's weekly meetings and publish it free of charge in the Academy's journal. However, she didn't take into consideration that she was a woman, a foreigner, and a liberal. When she announced her candidacy for the Academy, a sixty-six-year-old devout Catholic man was already in the race. The character of the contest abruptly changed. It became a sensational press campaign between, on the one hand, liberal, feminist groups and, on the other hand, nationalistic Catholics and anti–Semites who opposed the election of a foreign woman. Curie lost by one vote. This was a disappointment to Marie. She never again sought membership in the Academy and refused to publish her papers in its journal. The French Academy of Sciences refused to admit women until 1979.

Another unpleasant incident was the revelation that Marie might have had an affair with Paul Langevin who was a student and friend of Pierre. Langevin studied molecular structure of gases and did analyses of secondary emissions of X-ray from metals exposed to radiation. He was an outstanding physicist. Langevin and Marie were probably the only two French physicists who recognized the importance of quantum theory and Einstein's relativity theory. So it was natural that Marie appreciated and liked Paul. Unfortunately, most French scientists regarded Einstein's theories as Germanic and anti–French.

Langevin was five years younger than Marie, and he was a handsome and charming ladies' man. His marriage had been strained for years. His wife and her father wanted him to quit research and take a highly paid job in industry. The Curies and their friends, on the other hand, tried to save him for research. Unhappy with his marriage, he rented two rooms on the Rue du Banquier, a ten-minute walk from Curie's laboratory. In 1911 Marie began visiting him frequently and having lunch with him. They behaved like lovers as neighbors later told. So rumors spread quickly. Paul Langevin's wife, Jeanne, and her brother-in-law broke into the Paul's office and claimed to have secured some letters between Paul and Marie (clever pastiches assembled to incriminate her). Jeanne Langevin proceeded to secure a legal separation. "A Story of Love: Mme Curie and Professor Langevin" was released by *Le Journal*. Madame Curie's reputation was seriously damaged because the press reported that Marie was a Pole who had stolen a Frenchwoman's husband. Both Curie and the sciences were regarded as immoral and anti–French. The affair shook the University of Paris and the French government at the highest levels. Had it not been for a handful of close friends, Marie Curie would have left France and returned to Poland. It was not until Jeanne and Paul Langevin reached an out-of-court settlement on December 9, 1911 — with no mention of Marie Curie — that the scandal subsided.

Was there an affair between Paul Langevin and Marie Curie? No one will know for sure. In 1913, Langevin returned to his wife. Later, Paul Langevin's grandson married Marie Curie's granddaughter Hélène Joliot. Jeanne Langevin attended the wedding and held her tongue. Hélène Langevin-Joliot said, "I am more than eighty percent sure an affair occurred, but things were so different then, and people were so different. Conceivably, Langevin's apartment might have been for his work, to get out of the house, and to have an office."

After returning from Stockholm, Sweden, in 1911, Marie collapsed and was taken on a stretcher to a nursing home. Convinced that she had besmirched the Curie name, she insisted on using a pseudonym even to correspond with her daughter Irène.

She retreated once more into her shell, hiding her emotions. After coming out of the nursing home, she was devoted to building an institute for the study of radioactivity. By this time, Germany, Britain, and Denmark had already established physics institutes where groups of scientists could work together on common problems, but French physics professors still worked alone or with two or three students at the most. Marie Curie had begun talking with representatives of the University of Paris and the Pasteur Institute about a research center where scientists could do basic research in radioactivity, and physicians could apply that research to medical problems. A building for the institute was completed under her supervision. However, at that time, Curie was physically ill and emotionally exhausted. Her institute had a building but little more, not even a typewriter. She was not able to get financial support from government officials, industrialists, or philanthropists to do radioactivity research.

In August 1914 World War I broke out. Marie Curie realized immediately that X-ray would be invaluable for treating shrapnel and fracture wounds in frontline hospitals. She went to Paris and organized a mobile X-ray service. She filed a request with the minister of war for approval to begin work. She visited Parisian laboratories and wealthy women to ask for equipment, cars, and money. Her first vehicle was called a "petite Curie," which was ready for the Battle of the Marne in November 1914. By the end of the war, she had opened two hundred X-ray stations in French and Belgian battle zones and trained one hundred and fifty women technicians, including her daughter Irène. Her X-ray units examined more than one million soldiers.

Curie also began to collect the radon gas emitted from the radium. She sealed the gas in tiny glass tubes and shipped them to hospitals around the world for use against cancerous tumors. She was exhausted from this work and by that time had probably been exposed to more radiation than any other human being.

Despite her effort, the French government never recognized her patriotic work during the war. However, she learned that she could raise money, negotiate with the government, and run a large operation. She realized that she could use the Curie name and fame to promote a valuable cause.

After the war, Curie tried to convince the French public that a nation that does not invest in research is a nation on the decline. Unfortunately, the French economy was devastated by the war and postwar inflation. Her hope for financial support was extremely slim. Curie helped lobby government officials. She even changed her mind about scientists' patenting their discoveries, an issue that she strongly opposed before. Nevertheless, her efforts did not prevail.

In 1920 an important American woman showed up in her life. Mrs. Marie Mattingly Meloney Brown (generally known as Missy Meloney), the first woman with a seat in the press gallery of the United States Senate and editor of the *Delineator*, which was one of the largest women's magazines in the United States, came to see her in her office and understood Marie Curie's needs. Meloney arranged one of the largest fundraising campaigns the world had ever seen and raised one hundred thousand dollars to buy Curie a gram of radium. She also arranged a gala tour of the United States and honorary degrees from twenty universities for Marie Curie. President Warren Harding (1865–1923) gave Marie Curie a White House reception. When Marie, Irène, and Ève Curie arrived at the dock in New York City, they were greeted by cheering crowds, bands, banners, confetti, and frenzied newspaper reporters. Marie Curie was described in the *Scientific American* as "unassuming, plainly but neatly dressed, womanly and motherly in appearance.... She remains just plain Madame Curie, working for the good of humanity and for the expansion of scientific knowledge." Madame Curie was extremely famous and welcomed by Americans and proved to be a public relations dream. In 1929 she visited the United States again at the invitation of Meloney and collected enough money for a gram of radium for Poland. Meloney became Curie's close friend and confidante.

The glamour of the Curie name financed an international research center in France. She continued to do research, helping to untangle the process by which the radioactive elements decay into other elements. She organized, administered, and did fundraising for the institute. The Radium Institute became one of the world's leading centers for nuclear research. Many significant discoveries occurred in the institute. For example, Marguerite Perey (1909–1975) discovered francium, a new radioactive element; Salomon Rosenblum analyzed alpha rays; and Irène Curie and her husband, Frédérick Joliot-Curie, discovered artificial radioactivity. Curie reserved a certain number of positions for foreigners and women each year. In 1933 there were approximately 40 scientists at the institute, and seventeen of them were from foreign countries.

Curie also pushed for internationalization of physics. She helped Poland develop a radium institute and worked with the League of Nations committee on international publishing standards and student fellowships, helped establish the international standard for radium units, and donated radium and radon to researchers around the world.

At this stage of her life, Marie's health deteriorated rapidly. She had two cataract operations between 1920 and 1929. Cataracts are among the first symptoms of radiation damage. At one point, she was so blind that her lecture notes were printed two and a half inches high. She needed her daughter Irène to guide her to and from work. She tried to hide her condition and visited her ophthalmologist as Madame Carr.

The institute did not monitor the effect of radiation on health. Although several of Curie's lab workers died of anemia and leukemia during the 1920s, and Marie had anemia, tinnitus in her ears, and chronic exhaustion, still the effect of radiation on human health wasn't known. The institute did emphasize no smoking in the labs, changing lab coats frequently, and breathing fresh air outside whenever possible. Curie kept her health by breathing fresh air, swimming in the ocean, and doing mountain climbing. When an employee died, Curie thought it was because that employee did not get enough fresh air.

Although Curie was not healthy, she remained absolutely up to date on new developments in physics. She regularly attended conferences related to physics. And she kept her privacy. She destroyed almost all her personal papers including the correspondence between her and Paul Langevin, leaving only her love letters from Pierre, letters from a beau she had known during her student days, and a diary she had written after Pierre's death. There were testaments to the strength of the love that she and Pierre shared.

Toward the end of her life, she was still consumed with curiosity and a spirit of scientific adventure. She also organized an ordinary transition at the institute, arranging for André Debierne and then Irène to take over the directorship of the institute. She witnessed the discovery of artificial radioactivity by Irène and her husband, Frédérick Joliot-Curie. Their research had been under her supervision.

A few weeks before her death, she hiked alone partway up Mont Blanc to watch the sun set over the mountains. On July 4, 1934, she died of leukemia in a nursing home in Savoy, the French Alps, with her daughter Ève at her bedside. The ashes of Pierre and Marie Curie were transferred to the Panthéon on April 20, 1995.

The Curies lived a simple life. She and her husband Pierre lived in a three-room apartment without curtains, rugs, or excess furniture. She cared a lot about their gardens and views from their windows. She was not interested in housekeeping and did not spend time on anything that bored her. She spent most of her time studying, for which she had a strong sense of worth and respect. The Curies paid no attention to social calls that occupied too much time. They visited relatives and held a Sunday afternoon open house for friends and students. Their close friends were mostly scientists such as André Debierne, a chemist, physicist Jean Perrin (1870–1942) and his wife Aline, and Paul Langevin. Marie's interests were exclusively on sciences and family, but she was opinionated about political issues. The Curies were generally regarded as leftists and anticlerical republicans. They supported the government in spending more for education and scientific research that favored moral and material progress, disease prevention, better agricultural methods, electric tramways, street lighting, and the like. These viewpoints were contradictory to the viewpoints of the conservative Catholic groups in France.

In 1897 their daughter Irène (1897–1956) was born. Pierre's father, Eugene Curie, came to help while Marie continued to work. Eugene was a physician practicing homeopathy. He was extremely helpful to Mme. Curie. Both Marie's husband and her father in-law were supportive of her desire to continue studying, which was rather unusual for a working mother. At that time, she was one of two women in France working for a doctorate. She kept three notebooks — a baby's notebook, a laboratory notebook, and her household notebook — while she was pursuing her doctor's degree.

Isolating radium salts from tons of pitchblende had devastated the health of both Marie and Pierre. Not only did labor consume their physical energy, but they were also breathing the poisonous gas — radon emitted by radium. Marie had to commute weekly to Sèvres to give lectures at the teachers' training college for women. She suffered a miscarriage in 1903 after a long bicycle trip. Marie was always tired without being exactly ill, as Pierre told a friend.

The adverse effect of radiation on health was not known at that time. Marie liked to keep some radium salt glowing by her bedside. Pierre liked to carry a test tube of radium in his pocket to show friends. Pierre also performed medical experiments on his arm and showed that radium burns took months to heal. Marie and Pierre also loved to visit the shed at night to see the luminous test tube glowing like faint fairy lights. All these activities accelerated the deterioration of their health.

Both Marie and Pierre were devoted scientists, and they decided not to apply for patents on the industrial processes they devised for extracting radium salts from ore. They believed that research should be conducted for its own sake, not for any material rewards.

The death of Pierre was a big blow to Marie. She wrote, "What a terrible shock your poor head has felt, your poor head that I have so often caressed in my two hands.... We put you into the coffin Sunday morning, and I held your head up for this move. We kissed your cold face for the last time. Then a few periwinkles from the garden on the coffin and the little picture of me that you called 'the good little student' and that you loved. It is the picture that must go with you into the grave." Marie was close to a breakdown, but she kept her laboratory work going. She refused to accept a widow's pension. She insisted on being considered a scientist, not a helpless widow.

After the death of Pierre, Marie rarely spoke about Pierre to anyone; even late in life, she found it difficult to talk about him with her daughters. She reserved her deep private thoughts for the little gray exercise book. There she wrote, "My little Pierre, I want to tell you that the laburnum is in flower, the wisteria, the hawthorn and the iris are beginning. You should love it all. I would also like to tell you that they've given me your chair, and some imbeciles even congratulated me on it."

After the death of Pierre's father in 1910, she moved to a Parisian suburb and finally to a large apartment in central Paris. She disliked the rigid French school system. She organized a cooperative school for little Irène and her friends; she and other Sorbonne parents taught the class.

In 1913 she recovered and supervised the construction of her physics institute and went hiking in the Egadine with her daughters, some old friends including Albert Einstein and his young son. At this occasion, Einstein later recalled that Marie expressed her feeling mainly by grumbling.

Marie was very concerned with the health of their children and insisted on outdoor exercise for them. She took them backpacking and saw that they learned gymnastics, swimming, boating, horseback riding, and skiing as well as sewing and cooking. She built a summer house for August vacations in the Breton fishing village of L'Arcouest during the 1920s. She also built a house for herself on the Riviera because she enjoyed swimming herself. Despite her poor health and exposure to radioactivity, she remained strong. Her love of exercise and outdoor activity may have helped her avoid illnesses such as leukemia and other forms of cancer suffered by other colleagues working in the same conditions.

Despite Marie's formidable determination as a scientist, she often appeared timid and vulnerable to her daughters. By the time Ève was a young girl, her mother had pared their social lives to the minimum. When she had to face a large group, she suffered physically.

Marie Curie symbolized both the selfless pursuit of science and its humanitarian benefits. She was also imagined as the triumph of the lone individual against impossible odds. In France, she worked as though she were a fish swimming against a strong current. The Curies' refusal to patent their discoveries and their neglect by the French scientific establishment only fueled the legend.

In a biography of Marie Curie, her daughter Ève said, "I hope that the reader may constantly feel, across the ephemeral movement of one existence, what in Marie Curie was even more rare than her work or her life: the immovable structure of a character; the stubborn effort of an intelligence; the free immolation of a being that could give all and take nothing, could even receive nothing; and above all the quality of a soul in which neither fame nor adversity could change the exceptional purity."

* * *

It was noted that before Marie Curie received the Nobel Prize, the press had paid no attention to the science prize. The literature and peace awards received broad coverage, but the physics, chemistry, and medicine or physiology prizes were considered esoteric for the mass media. Marie Curie, however, made the science prizes so popular that the press never again ignored them.

Marie Curie's strong passion for knowledge and working for the good of humanity transmitted to her children. Her daughter Irène married Frédérick Joliot, and they were joint recipients of the Nobel Prize for chemistry in 1935 for the discovery of artificial radioactivity. Her other daughter Ève married the American diplomat H. R. Labouisse (1904–1987), who was a director of the United Nations Children's Fund and received on its behalf the Nobel Peace Prize in 1965. There were four Nobel Prize winners (Pierre, Marie, Irène and Frédérick) plus one on behalf of an important organization (Labouisse) associated with Marie Curie's family, which is an exceptional record in human history.

Marie Curie is a role model for women scientists. For example, Rosalyn Yalow (b.1921), a Nobel Prize laureate, said that she was greatly influenced by her example. There were many women who pursued science because of the example of Marie. However, her model was extremely hard for most women scientists to live up to. Most universities did not expect every male scientist to be an Albert Einstein but tended to expect women scientists to be a Marie Curie.

Behind every great individual is somebody, or a platoon of somebodies, a crowd of cheerleaders, sounding boards, tear-blotters, den mothers, den grandfathers, and so on. For Marie Curie, there were her parents, sisters, understanding husband Pierre, her father-in-law, colleagues, friends, and others who were important supporters. As we read the story of Marie Curie, we should remember that we can contribute much by numbering among a good platoon of somebodies for some extraordinary persons, even if we cannot be central examples of a successful life ourselves.

Radium was a very important element to be discovered. A piece of radium roughly the size of a penny is capable of producing approximately five hundred calories of heat every day for a thousand years. Peaceful utilization of nuclear energy will undoubtedly be an important part of human future civilization. The discovery of radium also led to the study of the nucleus, which brought the science into a different stage.

Marie Curie's scientific contribution stands in the same status as Galileo Galilei (1564–1642), Isaac Newton (1642–1727), and Albert Einstein (1879–1955). Yet she was also a great humanitarian as exemplified by her living style and numerous deeds helpful for humanity. She was a great woman. Her impact to human civilization both in science and humanity is beyond description.

Further Reading

Curie, Ève. (1937.) 2001. *Madame Curie: A Biography*. New York: Da Capo.

Ham, D. 2002/2003. Marie Sklodowska Curie: the woman who opened the nuclear age. *21st Century* (Winter 2002–2003): 30–68.

McGrayne, S. B. 1993. *Nobel Prize Women in Science: Their Lives, Struggles and Momentous Discoveries*. 2nd ed. Washington DC: Joseph Henry. 11–36.

Nobel Lectures, Physics 1901–1904. 1967. Amsterdam: Elsevier.

9

SARA JOSEPHINE BAKER
(1873–1945)

Physician and Pioneer Public Health Worker

The way to keep people from dying from disease, it struck me suddenly, was to keep them from falling ill. Healthy people don't die. It sounds like a completely witless remark, but at that time it was a startling idea. Preventive medicine had hardly been born yet and had no promotion in public health work.—Sara Josephine Baker (1873–1945)

Infectious diseases were a major concern for people before the 20th century as microbiology was in its infancy, and public health concepts and measures were generally lacking. Diarrhea, dysentery, pneumonia, smallpox, typhoid, cholera, influenza, and other diseases were major causes of death. In large cities such as New York and Boston, sanitation was generally inadequate, and in some cities was almost nonexistent. In New York City, one-third of all deaths were infants less than one year old. During the summer of 1902, in New York City's Hell's Kitchen district, 1,500 infants died of infectious diseases each week.

Preventive medicine was unknown. People would seek medical treatment only when they were sick. There were neither public health nurses nor large-scale public health programs or policies. However, things were slowly changing. Although female physicians were a rarity at the time, Sara Josephine Baker, one of them, was among the pioneers who instituted these changes.

Sara was born into a privileged family in Poughkeepsie, New York, on November 15, 1873. Her father was Orlando D. M. Baker, and her mother was Jennie Harwood (Brown) Baker. Sara was preparing for studies at Vassar by attending Misses Thomas' School for Young Ladies in Poughkeepsie. Unfortunately, her father died of typhoid fever when she was 16 years old. Against the will of her family and friends, in order to support her mother and family, she decided to study medicine. Getting into medical school was extremely difficult for women at that time since the only school that would accept women was the Woman's Medical College of New York Infirmary for Women and Children founded by Drs. Elizabeth (1821–1910) and Emily (1826–1910) Blackwell. The school closed in 1899 because Cornell University opened its medical college to women the same year.

After receiving her M.D. degree in 1898, Sara interned at the New England Hospital for Women and Children in Boston. She also worked at an outpatient clinic in one of Boston's worst slums, where she learned how poorly medical science was serving the crowded city population. She was so fed up with the filth of the hospital that she wrote, "Only the chorus of I-told-you-so that would have greeted me kept me from dropping it all and going home." Her first year of income from medical practice was $185.

At the turn of the 20th century, she began her life's work with the New York Department of Health as a medical inspector. Because she was a woman, she was given the terrible job of visiting slums. She went from home to home in the tenements of New York City to inspect for contagious diseases such as dysentery, smallpox, typhoid fever, etc. Probably no medical doctor today would be willing to do such a job. In her autobiography *Fighting for Life* (1939), Dr. Baker said, "I had let myself in for a really grueling ordeal. In my district, the heart of old Hell's Kitchen on the West Side, the heat, the smell, the squalor made it something not to be believed. I climbed stair after stair, knocked on door after door, met drunk after drunk, filthy mother after filthy mother, and dying baby after dying baby."

As a medical inspector, she examined children in public schools. She was allowed only one hour for every three schools. She could send home any child who was sick, but the truant officers were just as likely to send the sick child straight back to school. In an effort to curb the many health problems of school children, she established a city-wide school nursing program by organizing a team of 30 nurses to visit families door-to-door. Dr. Baker taught mothers of her district basic hygiene, nutrition, and ventilation. She established free milk stations, devising a simple baby formula by adding water, calcium carbonate and lactose to cow's milk. Not only did she invent a method of safely packaging and administering silver nitrate solution to newborn's eyes to prevent gonorrheal infection (caused by sexually transmitted *Neisseria gonorrhoeae*) and subsequent blindness, she also designed baby clothes that were safe and convenient for the newborn and small babies.

Her program worked so successfully that cases of head lice and trachoma (caused by *Chlamydia trachomatis*), which had been extremely prevalent in schools at the time, dropped to nearly zero. The death rates among infants in the city of her district decreased from 1,500 per week to 300 per week in the summer of 1908. Soon after, the Division of Child Hygiene, later known as the Bureau of Child Hygiene, was established, and Dr. Sara Josephine Baker was appointed its chief.

When the Bureau of Child Hygiene was formed, a petition was signed by more than 30 Brooklyn physicians and sent to the mayor demanding that the Bureau be abolished because "it was ruining medical practice by its results in keeping babies well." Dr. Baker told the mayor that the letter was a compliment to the bureau.

Dr. Baker created a program considered controversial at the time. It was the Little Mother Leagues, in which eight- to nine-year-old girls were trained to take care of younger children while the mothers went to work earning money to buy food. Many protested the Leagues were "enslaving the young girls so their mothers could be irresponsible, go to the movies, or get drunk."

One of the diseases common in Dr. Baker's day was typhoid fever, which is caused by *Salmonella typhi*. Before antibiotics were available, the mortality rate from typhoid fever was about 20 percent, but a substantial number of recovered patients become chronic carriers, harboring the pathogen in their gallbladder and continuing to shed the pathogen and spread the disease. A historical example of a typhoid fever carrier was "Typhoid Mary" (1868–1938). Her story was a good lesson of epidemiology and public health. One of the famous professional tasks in Dr. Baker's life was to help track down Typhoid Mary.

Mary Mallon was an Irish immigrant who earned her living as a cook. In 1901 Mary was working for a family who had a visitor who came down with typhoid fever. One month later Mary and several laundresses developed the same disease. In 1902 after she recovered, she began working for another family. Two weeks after she started working in that family, the laundresses and six members of that family contracted the disease. Mary left that house. In 1903 Mary worked as a cook in a household in Ithaca, New York, and was believed to have started a waterborne typhoid outbreak that spread widely, killing 1,300 people. In 1904 Mary moved to a house in Long Island; within three weeks, four servants developed typhoid fever. In 1906 Mary moved again and within a week six people in her new employer's house fell ill with typhoid. Two weeks later, Mary, having been suspected to be the source of infection, fled to another family. After another two weeks, the family's laundress developed typhoid fever.

In 1906 Dr. George A. Soper (1870–1948), a military physician, was hired by the New York City Health Department to investigate the outbreak of typhoid in Long Island. He became suspicious about the possible link of Mary with the typhoid outbreak and decided to track Mary down. In 1907 Mary used a false name to work as a cook again for a family in New York

City. Two months after her arrival, two household members developed typhoid. Mary immediately left but was tracked down. Dr. Baker was sent to collect specimens for testing to determine whether Mary was a carrier of the pathogen. What happened was described in the book *Women Life Scientists: Past, Present, and Future* (1997): "On her first visit, Baker had the door slammed in her face. The next day, when she returned with several policemen, Mary answered the door and again tried to slam it shut, but a policeman's foot was in the door. Mary ran into the house and could not be found in a search of the house. But looking out the rear window, Dr. Baker noticed a chair against the fence and footprints in the snow. Mary was found next door hiding in a closet." Mary was confined to a hospital for nearly three years, then released on a promise never to work as a cook again. She promptly disappeared. More than five years later, she resurfaced, was captured, and was sent to North Brother Island, where she remained confined until her death in 1938.

With initial reluctance, Dr. Baker later became a feminist and a suffragette. She struggled to get political recognition for the fact that women are human beings with the same rights as men. She participated in the first suffrage parade that occurred on Fifth Avenue. She was a member of the delegation that visited President Woodrow Wilson (1856–1924) in the White House to request his official endorsement of the Nineteenth Amendment, which gave women the right to vote. The text of the Nineteenth Amendment is: "Section 1. The right of citizens of the United States to vote shall not be denied or abridged by the United States or by any State on account of sex. Section 2. Congress shall have power to enforce this article by appropriate legislation."

Later Dr. Baker served as an officer, consultant, or board member for a number of professional associations including the influential Heterodoxy that served as a network for women during the early part of the 20th century in the United States. She was a member of the board and consulting pediatrician of Clinton (New Jersey) Reformatory for Women and a member of the Health Commission. She was the honorary president of the Children's Welfare Federation Trustees of the New York Infirmary for Women and Children. She was president and founding member of the American Child Health Association. She was also president of the American Hygiene Association and the American Medical Women's Association. Additionally, she was the first woman to serve the League of Nations in an official capacity. She published five books and over 200 articles during her professional career including her autobiography, *Fighting for Life*, published in 1939.

Dr. Baker lived in a time when women were not considered equal to men professionally and socially, especially in the field of medicine. She had a hard time getting into medical school because most medical schools did not admit women. The only medical school admitting women was the Women's Medical College of the New York Infirmary for Women and Children. Because of the anti-female prejudice, she was assigned to the most undesirable job when she was employed at the New York Department of Health, visiting door to door in the slums to check for contagious diseases. Even after her success in reducing infant sickness and mortality, she faced jealousy from male physicians. Some of them resented the fact that a female physician was in charge of a city bureau. When she was first appointed director of the division, six male physicians resigned because they considered it a disgrace to work for a woman. She had to persuade them to try it for a month. During her tenure in that position, she often faced pressure to be removed from her position because of her gender. There was considerable pressure to remove her in 1919 but fortunately, she received great public support from the local press and from mothers who marched to the mayor's office to protest her possible dismissal.

Dr. Baker had been invited to be a guest lecturer at the New York University Medical School. When she delivered a lecture to students for the Doctor of Public Health degree, she summarized her experience as follows:

"I stood in a well with tiers of seats rising all around me — and the seats were filled with unruly, impatient, hard boiled young men. I looked them over and opened my mouth to begin the lecture. Instantly, before a syllable could be heard, they began to clap thunderously, deafeningly, grinningly, and pounding their palms together."

Dr. Baker would roar with laughter to save face. But at the end of the lecture, she was warmly applauded. This happened every time for the 15 years she lectured.

Because she was a woman, despite her great accomplishments, Dr. Baker was never awarded a doctorate in public health.

*   *   *

Just as the pioneers planted trees so that people later could enjoy the coolness of their shade, Dr. Baker planted the seed that helped cultivate the women's movement so that women in the future could aspire to equality with men. She struggled for the women's right to professional competence. It is interesting to note that although she was placed in the most terrible job when she first reported to work at the New York City Department of Health, she accomplished a great deal on that job and left human beings with a huge legacy that we treasure today. She turned the circumstances resulting from gender discrimination into something of benefit for herself and for all human beings.

Dr. Albert Einstein (1879–1955) said, "Try to be a person of value, not a person of success." Dr. Baker was a woman of value. Even as a child, Dr. Baker's life suggested that she would be great. Her characteristics in childhood were indicative of the magnitude of her greatness, which she would eventually develop. Her compassion, persistence, and empathy were evident. In her autobiography, she said:

> My impulse to try to do things about hopeless situations appears to have cropped up first when I was about six years old, and it should be pointed out that the method I used was characteristically direct. I was all dressed up for some great occasion — a beautiful white lacy dress with a blue sash and light blue silk stockings and light blue kid shoes — and inordinately vain about it. While waiting for Mother to come down, I wandered out in front of the house to sit on the horse block and admire my self and hope that some one would come along and see me in all my glory.
>
> Presently a spectator did arrive — a little colored girl about my size but thin and peaked and hungry looking, wearing only a ragged old dress the color of ashes. I have never seen such dumb envy in any human being's face before or since. Child that I was, I could not stand it, it struck me right over the heart. I could not bear the idea that I had so much and she had so little. So I got down off the horse block and took off every stitch I had on, right down to the blue shoes that were the joy of my infantile heart and gave everything, underwear and all to the little black girl. I watched her as she scampered away, absolutely choked with bliss. Then I walked back into the house, completely naked, wondering why I had done it and how to explain my inexplicable conduct. Oddly enough both Father and Mother seemed to understand pretty well what had gone in my mind. They were fine people, my Father and Mother.

Sara Josephine Baker never married. She retired in 1923. Beginning in 1935, she stayed in a house with Louise Pearce (1885–1959), another well known female medical doctor, and Ida A. R. Wylie (1885–1959), a well known writer, in Trevanna Farm, Skillmann, New Jersey. Another companion was Florence Laighton. Great spirits seem to attract each other. Dr. Baker died on February 22, 1945, at the Trevanna Farm.

Was it necessary for those pioneer women to sacrifice family life in order to accomplish extraordinary endeavors? Could they also have enjoyed family life as well as their male counterparts while they were pursuing their careers?

The incident of Typhoid Mary also deserves more thinking. Was Mary Mallon the only person who spread the disease in her time? The answer is apparently no. Mary Mallon was singled out to be apprehended and isolated on Manhattan's North Brother Island, where she died 23 years later. However, other typhoid carriers — male — were let go in a few days.

Gender discrimination, personal rights, and communicable infectious diseases are still serious modern maladies for the human race. The contributions of Dr. S. J. Baker and her life experiences deserve to remain in our memory.

Further Reading

Baker, Sara Josephine. 1939. *Fight for Life*. Huntington NY: R. E. Krieger.

Matyas, Karen Lakes, and Ann E. Haley-Oliphant. 1997. *Women Life Scientists: Past, Present, and Future*. Bethesda MD: American Physiological Society.

Tortora, G. J., B. R. Funke, and C. L. Case. 2003. *Microbiology: An Introduction*. 8th ed. San Francisco: Benjamin Cummings Pearson. 714–715.

10

ALICE CATHERINE EVANS
(1881–1975)

Researcher in Bacteriology and
Promoter of Pasteurization of Milk

Alice Evans was a pioneer both as a scientist and as a woman leader. She discovered that drinking unpasteurized milk was the major way of contracting brucellosis (undulant fever). Cow milk was easily contaminated with *Brucella abortus* from cattle, whereas sheep or goat milk was contaminated with *B. melitensis*. (Other Brucella species include *B. canis*, which can cause brucellosis in dogs, and *B. suis*, which can cause brucellosis in swine. These species are not major concerns for human health.) Evans fought persistently for the pasteurization of milk before the milk was sold to the market. She eventually won the battle by law. The milk we buy today has been pasteurized, stopping people from contracting undulant fever from drinking milk.

Evans was also a leader. In 1928 she became the first woman president of the Society of American Bacteriologists (now the American Society for Microbiology, ASM, which counts more than 40,000 members). Her work had a major impact on microbiology in the United States and the world.

Alice Catherine Evans was born on January 29, 1881, in the Welsh town of Neath, Pennsylvania. Her grandfather immigrated from Wales and settled in Pennsylvania in 1831. Her father was William Howell, and her mother was Anne Evans. William Howell was a surveyor, teacher, farmer, and Civil War veteran. Anne Evans migrated from Wales at the age of 14.

Alice Evans received her primary education at the local district school in Neath. She continued to study at the Susquehanna Institute at Towanda, Pennsylvania. Unable to afford college tuition, she became a grade school teacher. After teaching for four years, she enrolled in a two-year program in natural science at the College of Agriculture of Cornell University. It was a tuition-free program designed to help teachers in rural areas to develop an appreciation of nature. Her teachers included G. Wilder (1862–1925), who taught vertebrate zoology, and the very famous entomologist Dr. John Henry Comstock (1849–1931).

Evans never returned to teaching; her life path had been significantly changed. She continued her education at Cornell University and obtained a B.S. degree in agriculture in 1908. Strongly recommended by Professor William A. Stocking of Cornell, she was offered a scholarship at the University of Wisconsin, where she studied under the supervision of Professor E. G. Hastings (1872–1953). In 1910 she obtained a master's degree in bacteriology. Dr. Elmer V. McCollum (1879–1967), who taught chemistry of nutrition and later discovered vitamin A and D, encouraged her to continue to enroll in a Ph.D. program. Because of financial and physical strains, she did not pursue further studies at that time.

She was offered a research position by Professor Hastings with the Dairy Division of the Department of Agriculture at the University of Wisconsin. At the time, several state agricultural experiment stations were collaborating with the United States Department of Agriculture (USDA) in cooperative research. On July 1, 1910, she began investigating an improved method of cheese making. As she worked, she took one course each year to fill gaps in her education. In 1913 she moved with the Dairy Division of the Department of Agriculture to Washington, D.C., and worked as a bacteriological technician in the Bureau of Animal Industry, USDA. Alice Evans was the first woman scientist to hold a permanent appointment at the USDA. Fortunately, she found that her immediate supervisors, B. G. Rawl, chief of the division, and Lore A. Rogers, in charge of research, had a favorable attitude toward women in science.

Her job was to isolate the contaminants of raw cow's milk. At that time, the general belief was that the freshly drawn milk was quite healthy. This project was studied by a team: William Mansfield Clark (1884–1964), chemist; Alice Evans, bacteriologist; and Lore A. Rogers, project leader. Clark later became renowned for developing an accurate method of measuring pH.

Malta fever (also called Mediterranean fever or undulant fever) caused by *Brucella melitensis* (originally called *Micrococcus melitensis*; Meyer and Shaw renamed it *Brucella melitensis* in 1920) was isolated by David Bruce (1855–1931) in 1886. In 1905 T. Zammit found that goat milk was the disseminating vehicle of Malta fever. Evans also discovered that a bacterium in the raw milk was responsible for human undulant fever. The bacterium isolated from cow's milk was similar to the one that caused spontaneous abortion in cows (*Brucella abortus*). The bacterium isolated from the milk and the one that caused abortion produced similar effects in guinea pigs. Evans demonstrated that the two organisms could be differentiated by an agglutinin absorption test. It was clear to her that raw cow's milk had the potential of transmitting undulant fever. However, when Evans presented her findings to the Society of American Bacteriologists in 1917, they were received with skepticism, partly because she was a woman and partly because she did not have a Ph.D. degree. Despite her insistence that pasteurization of milk was necessary before selling to the market, she received no response. In those days the general public of America did not believe that raw milk would transmit diseases.

In 1918 Dr. George McCoy (b.1876) asked Evans to join the U.S. Public Health Service, of which he was director. She joined a group of doctors who were striving to improve antiserum production used in treatment of epidemic meningitis, one of the dreaded diseases of World War I, with a fatality rate of more than 50 percent. Because of her involvement in this research, she was unable to continue her studies on milk. However, Evans' findings attracted world attention, and the controversy on the significance of *Brucella abortus* in milk continued.

One of the most well-known scientists opposing the idea that brucellae in cow's milk might cause human diseases was Theobald Smith (1859–1934), who published reports in 1919 and again in 1925, disagreeing with the premise that the brucellae in milk might be hazardous to health. Although Smith recognized brucellae in milk as an indicator of bovine infection, he rejected the assumption that consumption of such milk was hazardous to human health. In 1925 when Dr. Smith learned that Evans was to become a member of the National Research Council's Committee on Infectious Abortion, he declined to become chairman of the committee because he had a conflicting opinion on the dissemination of undulant fever by milk.

Meanwhile, cases of human brucellosis caused by drinking infected cow's milk were found in southern Rhodesia and Britain, and African medical journals reported many cases of brucellosis in humans contracted from infected cows.

Dr. Smith continued for some time to raise valid questions about the epidemiology of brucellosis, based on the scarcity of known human infections. However, evidence of undulant fever of bovine origin had come from nine European countries and from Palestine, Canada, and Denmark. Furthermore, in 1922 Evans herself contracted brucellosis, and *Brucella melitensis* was shown to be the etiological agent. Her condition was chronic, bothering her off and on for about 23 years. Concomitant with her illness, she developed a hypersensitivity to brucellar antigens.

The symptoms of brucellosis were varied and very similar to those of influenza, typhoid fever, tuberculosis, and rheumatism. For this reason it was not often correctly diagnosed. However, Evans made effort to document cases of the undulant fever in the United States and South Africa. She also surveyed the different parts of the U.S. to determine the number of infected

cows from which raw milk was sold and the number of chronic cases resulting from the milk. The problem of chronic brucellosis became widespread in
the United States. There were many incidences of death of farmers' children
caused by their drinking contaminated milk. Evans strongly recommended
that milk be pasteurized before consumption. Eventually, public health officials
finally began to recognize the need for milk pasteurization in 1930.

Evans felt that the opposition to her discovery was partly due to sexual
discrimination. Now we appreciate Evans' persistence in fighting with courage and with strong scientific evidence, and we are grateful that, thanks to
her efforts, pasteurization of milk is presently mandatory in every state.

In 1928 Evans was elected president of the Society of American Bacteriologists. Not only was she the first woman president of this large society but
her administrative skill was also highly praised. In 1936 Evans returned to a
study of chronic brucellosis. She set up and coordinated a project employing
field investigations in different cities where a large percentage of milk was still
consumed raw. She also surveyed bovine brucellosis as a part of the program
of eradication of the cattle disease.

In the course of her work at the National Institutes of Health (NIH),
she also researched meningococci with Dr. Sara Branham (1888–1962) and
studied clostridial toxins with Dr. Ida Benstan. Around 1939 Evans began an
investigation of immunity to streptococcal infections. At the time, there were
some 30 known types of streptococci. When she retired in 1945, 46 types had
been characterized.

Evans took advantage of numerous opportunities for travel. In 1930 she
was an American delegate to the First International Congress of Bacteriology
held at the Pasteur Institute in Paris, France. During the meeting, she had
the chance to meet world renowned microbiologists including Dr. Lydia Rabi-
nowich, known for her work on tuberculosis; Dr. Azzo Azzi, editor of an Italian microbiological review journal; Professor Hans Olaf Bang of Copenhagen,
son of Bernhard Lauritis Bang (1848–1932), discoverer of the causal organism of contagious abortion (brucellosis) in cattle; Dr. John C. G. Ledingham
(1875–1944), director of the Lister Institute in London; Dr. Jules Bordet
(1870–1961), a Nobel Prize laureate and director of the Pasteur Institute in
Brussels; Dr. Albert Calmette (1863–1933), inventor of BCG vaccine for
tuberculosis; and Dr. William H. Park (1863–1939) of New York. She took
advantage of this trip to travel to many parts of France and other European
countries.

She also attended the Second International Congress of Bacteriology in
London in 1936. In this meeting, she had the chance to meet contemporary
distinguished microbiologists including Dr. Fred Griffith (1877–1941), dis-

coverer of bacterial transformation; Sir Weldon Dalrymple-Champneys (–1941), expert on brucellosis; and Dr. John Eyre, who had some three decades earlier been a member of the commission headed by Dr. David Bruce, who investigated the "Mediterranean Fever." After the meeting, she traveled to Europe and visited Delft, Netherlands, where she was well received by Dr. Albert Jan Kluyver (1888–1956) and his guest, Dr. C. B. Van Niel (1897–1985), by then located in California. They were all pioneer microbiologists. In Belgium, she visited Professor Van de Velde, a renowned biochemist. Those trips were so memorable to Evans that she left a record of impressions in an addendum to her memoirs.

Evans received many honors in her life. In 1934 she received an honorary M.D. from Women's Medical College (now Medical College of Pennsylvania). In 1936 she received an honorary D.Sc. from Wilson College, and in 1948 she received an honorary D.Sc. from the University of Wisconsin. She was also made an honorary member of the American Society for Microbiology in 1975.

Dr. Evans had an independent spirit and uncompromising integrity as evidenced by her life in investigating brucellosis transmitted by contaminated milk. Her perseverance in investigation led to changes in public health practice that saved many lives.

She also had a strong interest in young people and minorities. Through the auspices of the Washington Branch of the American Association of University Women, she set up a tuition fellowship for Federal City College in Washington, D.C.

Dr. Evans' insistence on principle can also be seen in another incident. At the age of 85 when she applied for Medicare, according to the law, Evans was required to sign a form disclaiming Communist affiliation. Evans refused to do it because she thought that signing the form would be a denial of her constitutional right. She never signed and the form was processed without her signature.

Evans spent her last years in Goodwin House in Alexandria, Virginia, and following a stroke, she passed away on September 5, 1975, at age 94. She never married.

* * *

Pasteurization of milk is a necessity in our modern world. With Evans' persistent effort we drink safer milk, and therefore, we live longer and may be healthier than our ancestors. Because the process of pasteurization bears the name of its creator, we remember the contribution of Louis Pasteur. Sadly, however, Alice Evans' contribution is much less recognized.

Fortunately, in memory of Dr. Evans's work, the American Society for Microbiology Committee on the Status of Women in Microbiology established the Alice C. Evans Award to recognize individuals who made major contributions toward the full participation of women in microbiology. The first award was given in 1983 to Dr. Frederick C. Neidhardt. This author has the honor of serving on the Awards Committee of the American Academy of Microbiology (2004–2007) responsible for the nomination of the candidates for this award.

Further Reading

Burns, Virginia Law. 1993. *Gentle Hunter: A Biography of Alice C. Evans, Bacteriologist*. Laingsburg MI: Enterprise.

Colwell, R. R. 1999. Alice C. Evans. *Yale Journal of Biology and Medicine* 72: 349–356.

Colon, Diana M. 1997. Alice Catherine Evans (1881–1975). In *Women in the Biological Sciences: A Biobibliographic Sourcebook*. Edited by Louise S. Grinstein, Carol A. Biermann, and Rose K. Rose. Westport CT: Greenwood. 163–169.

O'Hern, E. M. 1973. Alice Evans, pioneer microbiologist. *American Society of Microbiology News* 39: 573–578.

11

LOUISE PEARCE
(1885–1959)

Leader in Research on Both
African Sleeping Sickness and Syphilis

Trypanosomiasis (African sleeping sickness) is a protozoan disease that affects the nervous system. It is caused by trypanosomes of the brucei group: *Trypanosoma gambiense* and *T. rhodesiense*. These flagellates are injected by the bite of tsetse fly (glossina). In 1907, an epidemic of sleeping sickness occurred in Uganda with a terrible death toll. Winston Churchill (1874–1965) described Uganda as a "beautiful garden of death" during the epidemic. Today, the disease still affects about one million people in central and east Africa, and about 20,000 new cases are reported each year. The symptoms include decrease in physical activity and mental acuity. If the disease is untreated, the infected person goes into a coma and eventually dies.

Dr. Louise Pearce was well known for her contribution to the cure of trypanosomiasis and earned the nickname of "a magic bullet for African Sleeping Sickness." She traveled to the Congo to conduct field tests to determine the effectiveness of the drug tryparsamide developed by the Rockefeller Research Institute, now Rockefeller University. She wiped out trypanosomiasis in animals and eventually put the medicine into practical use for humans.

Dr. Pearce also contributed greatly to the study of syphilis by developing an animal model. She discovered the Brown-Pearce tumor, the first transplantable tumor in rabbits, which was used in cancer research laboratories worldwide.

Louise Pearce was born on March 5, 1885, in Winchester, Massachusetts. Her father was Charles Ellis Pearce, a cigar and tobacco dealer. Her mother was Susan Elizabeth Hoyt. She had a younger brother named Robert Pearce, who later became an attorney in New York City. Little is known about her childhood. Her family moved to California sometime before 1900 and lived on a ranch in the Los Angeles area. Her family finances were sufficient for her to attend the Girls' Collegiate School in Los Angeles from 1900 to 1903. She then attended Stanford University in Palo Alto and graduated with an A.B. degree in Physiology and Histology in 1907, a truly pioneering achievement for a woman in those days.

After graduation, Louise moved to Boston to work for two years as an instructor in embryology and as an assistant in histology for Boston University School of Medicine. In 1908 she was offered a scholarship to attend the Women's Medical College of Pennsylvania in Philadelphia, but she declined the offer in order to attend the Johns Hopkins University School of Medicine. Louise Pearce obtained her M.D. degree in 1912, graduating third in her class. She followed in the footsteps of Dr. Florence Sabin (1871–1953), who was a well-known American anatomist. After graduation, she served as an intern at Johns Hopkins Hospital.

In 1913, Dr. Pearce was on the staff of the Phipps Psychiatric Clinic at Johns Hopkins Hospital. Although she had a prestigious position, she wasn't happy as a house officer; she wanted to have a laboratory research position. Therefore, she wrote to Dr. Simon Flexner (1863–1946), director of the Rockefeller Institute in New York City, to apply for a research position. Dr. Flexner was impressed by her excellent academic record and wanted to include a woman on the institute's scientific staff. He hired her as an assistant fellow at the Rockefeller Institute to work directly under him. She worked closely with Dr. Wade Hampton Brown (1878–1942), who spent his life working on the susceptibility or resistance of hosts to infection. They built animal models for syphilis and trypanosomiasis in rabbits as a part of their research. In this capacity, Dr. Pearce focused her research on trypanosomiasis. Her work had a great impact on the fight against this terrible human malady, and she became well known in the scientific community.

At about that time, trypanosomiasis plagued many African countries, and the Rockefeller Institute was involved in the search for a solution. Salvarsan, an arsenic compound, was discovered by Paul Ehrlich (1854–1915) to be effective for the treatment of syphilis. This stimulated scientists to develop other drugs. Dr. Flexner asked his colleagues at the Rockefeller Institute to try to find other arsenical compounds for use to treat trypanosomiasis. In 1919 Walter Jacobs and Michael Heidelberger found a compound called tryparsamide, which was tested by Drs. Pearce and Brown and found to be highly effective in destroying the infectious agents of trypanosomiasis in animals. A field trial on humans was urgently needed. In 1920 there was a severe outbreak of trypanosomiasis in the Congo (a Belgian colony at that time). The Rockefeller Institute intended to send Dr. Brown to the Congo to test the new compound, but Dr. Brown, a family man, wasn't enthusiastic about going there. Dr. Pearce, however, was attracted to the adventure of field research and volunteered to go alone to Leopoldville, Congo, to test the new drug. Dr. Pearce studied the effect of each dose of tryparsamide on more than seventy patients and observed the complete eradication of the parasite in the blood and nervous system within a few weeks of the treatment with no side effects.

Dr. Pearce's contribution made her well known internationally. Her work impressed the Belgian officials, and she was awarded the Ancient Order of the Crown in 1921. She was elected a member of the Belgian Society of Tropical Medicine and every year, from 1921 to 1939, she made a trip to Europe either to attend a scientific meeting or to take part in other activities.

After her success in Africa, she returned to the Rockefeller Institute in New York and was promoted to associate member in 1923. Her research accomplishments should really have qualified her to be promoted to a full member. However, because of the Depression at that time, the Research Institute was short of funds and she wasn't granted such a promotion, which would have given her the freedom to pursue research goals separately from her colleague, Dr. Wade H. Brown. Sadly, she remained as an associate member of the institute until her retirement. She continued her research on syphilis and tested tryparsamide's ability to reach the central nervous system.

In 1924 she went to Africa again to conduct large trials. She confirmed that tryparsamide was effective in humans, but that large doses used in the treatment of advanced cases resulted in damaged vision and occasionally blindness. She urged her departmental head, Dr. Flexner, to end these heroic trials, and she began the widespread treatment of the afflicted patients. She served as representative for the Rockefeller Institute and as a contact for the physicians conducting trials in her absence. She also was a medical consulting delegate for the International Conference on Christian Missions in Africa in 1926. Her work in Africa was published in 1930 as *The Treatment of Human Trypanosomiasis with Tryparsamide: A Critical Review.*

In collaboration with Dr. Brown, Dr. Pearce also made a lot of progress on the study of syphilis. The syphilis infection of the nervous system was a hopeless situation in those days. Drs. Pearce and Brown worked on an experimental model in rabbits. They thought that tryparsamide, which was capable of penetrating the brain and spinal cord, might be able to kill the syphilis spirochetes in the nervous system. They did prove that the drug was effective, and even more effective in combination with an artificial fever. Tryparsamide in combination with artificial fever was an accepted treatment of syphilis until the availability of penicillin, which was discovered by Alexander Fleming (1881–1955) in 1928.

Dr. Pearce studied the disease diligently. She did some comparison of the blood components of normal and syphilis-infected animals. She also studied the effect of co-infection of syphilis spirochaete with a vaccinia virus. In 1922 while observing syphilis-infected rabbits, she and Dr. Brown discovered that one rabbit had a malignant tumor of the scrotum that could be successfully propagated to other rabbits. This was followed by an extensive study of the factors that would affect the susceptibility of the host to the implanted cells. She tested the effect of tumor presence on polio infection and on blood composition of the infected animals and the effects of seasons and the exposure to light on normal and tumor-infected rabbits. Also, in collaboration with Dr. Thomas Rivers (1887–1963), she conducted a series of experiments attempting to find a correlation between virus infection and tumor formation. Eventually the well-characterized rabbit tumor she and Dr. Brown had discovered was called the Brown-Pearce tumor and became a popular material for the study of cancer.

In 1931 Dr. Pearce was invited to be a visiting professor of syphilology by Peiping Union Medical College in Peking (now called Beijing), China. She brought along 125 rabbits to China in order to compare the Western version of syphilis with an "Oriental " strain. She worked in China from November 1931 until May 1932 and discovered that what had appeared to be two different strains of syphilis proved to be the same spirochete on two different species of rabbits. During this time, civil wars were raging in China. Japan invaded Manchuria, and China was in turmoil. Many of Dr. Pearce's fellow visiting professors were sent to Shanghai. Her research work was hindered.

Upon her return from China, Brown and Pearce's experiments were seriously set back by a deadly smallpox-like disease of their rabbit colonies. However, with the collaboration of Drs. Paul Rosahn (b. 1903), Harry Greene (b. 1904), and C. K. Hu, they proved the disease was viral in nature, and that the rabbit was an excellent model for the study of human smallpox. They investigated extensively the epidemiology, immune reactions, and susceptibility of rabbits to different diseases. This valuable information was published in the *Proceedings of the Society for Experimental Biology and Medicine*, 30:894–896 (1932–1933).

In 1935 Dr. Brown's research group including Dr. Pearce was asked to move from New York City to a facility of the Rockefeller Institute in Princeton. The new building provided more room for the rabbit colonies and decreased the cost of maintaining those colonies. However, Dr. Brown soon became ill and was forced to downsize his activities. This had a negative effect on Dr. Pearce's research. Following the death of Dr. Brown in 1942, Dr. Pearce finished his experiments and published the data.

Dr. Brown's main interest was to see how inherited disorders would make an animal more susceptible to diseases. The rabbit colonies displayed several inherited syndromes, such as a rickets-like forepaw malformation, excessively dense bones, a complex disorder that included premature aging, early death, and achondroplasia.

In 1947 Dr. Pearce was asked to conclude her experimentation, and she was granted three years' full pay to write up her experimental results, followed by half pay until retirement in 1951. Dr. Pearce continued to write articles until her death and her assistant, Margaret Dunham, finished and submitted the last two articles after her death.

In addition to doing research, Dr. Pearce also actively participated in many other meaningful activities. From 1921 to 1928, she served as a trustee of the New York Infirmary for Women and Children, a women's medical college established by Dr. Elizabeth Blackwell (1821–1910). She was a member of the Executive Board of the American Medical Women's Association (1935–36) and an honorary member of the editorial board of its journal. Dr. Pearce also served on the Committee to Award International Fellowships for the International Federation of University Women from 1938 to 1946 and served as second vice president (1950–1953) of this federation.

In addition, she served as a trustee for Princeton Hospital from 1940 to 1944. She also was a member of the Board of Corporators of the Women's Medical College of Pennsylvania from 1941 to 1959.

Dr. Pearce was supportive of women's rights and a great promoter of women's education. In 1946, she became president of the Women's Medical College of Pennsylvania and held that position till her retirement in 1951. She presided over the college's centenary celebration in 1950, which was a big memorable event for the college. She served as director in the American Association for University Women between 1945 to 1951, and as committee chairman for International Associations (1946–1951).

In addition to the Ancient Order of the Crown in 1921 of Belgium, Pearce was awarded the King Leopold Prize of $10,000 in 1953. Dr. Pearce was elected to the Royal Society of Tropical Medicine and Hygiene in 1924. She was also appointed a member of the scientific advisory council of the American Social Hygiene Association (1921–1941) and was on the National Research Council from 1931 to 1933. She became a member of the Pathology Society of Great Britain and Ireland in 1932.

Dr. Pearce also received honorary doctorates from several colleges including Wilson College, Beaver College, Bucknell College, Skidmore College, and the Women's Medical College of Pennsylvania. She also received the Elizabeth Blackwell Award from the New York Infirmary in 1951.

Dr. Louise Pearce never married or had children, and we have little information about her personal life. However, she had an active social life and numerous professional friends. In 1935 when she was asked to move to Princeton, New Jersey, her friends Dr. Ida A. R. Wylie (1885–1959) and Dr. Sara Josephine Baker (1873–1945) decided to move from their apartment in New York City to join Pearce in sharing a house, which was purchased by Dr. Wylie in Skillmann Montgomery Township, New Jersey. Dr. Wylie was a British novelist, and well known for *The Daughter of Brahma*, which was published in 1912. She also published her autobiography, *My Life with George*, in 1940. Dr. Baker was a physician and later the first chief of the Department of Child Hygiene at the New York City Department of Health. Dr. Baker was a pioneer in public health education. Drs. Wylie, Baker and Pearce were active in the women's rights movement. They did much to advance the cause of women, particularly in the fields of medicine and science.

They lived in Trevanna Farm house just outside Princeton. It was a big house that could accommodate the three women, some maids, and Wylie's several dogs. The three professional women supported each other in their careers. When Dr. Baker retired in 1923, she assumed responsibility for running the household. With Dr. Baker and their servants to manage the household concerns, Wylie and Pearce were able to concentrate on their work. They would always vacation together, either at Martha's Vineyard in Massachusetts or in Europe. They also attended parties given by Wylie's publisher. Baker died in 1945, and Pearce and Wylie continued to live at the farm. Dr. Pearce fell ill on an ocean liner returning from a trip to Europe. She died on August 9, 1959, in New York City. Dr. Wylie died three months afterward, and the bulk of her estate was donated to the Women's Medical College of Pennsylvania in Pearce's memory.

* * *

Dr. Pearce was a pioneer with a great spirit, who cared not for personal interest, but for the healthiness of humanity. She bravely traveled to the Congo to conduct field trials of the effectiveness of the drug tryparsamide to African sleeping sickness patients. Similarly she also bravely traveled to China to pursue syphilis study. She totally ignored personal inconveniences and risks to work for the interest of mankind. Her great spirit not only saved human physical lives, it enlightened humanity as well.

Further Reading

Baumann, F. 1960. Memorial to Louise Pearce, M.D. (1885–1959). *Journal of the American Medical Women's Association* (August): 793.

Fay, M. 1961. Louise Pearce, 5th March 1885–9th August 1959. *Journal of Pathology and Bacteriology* **82**: 542–551.

Fulton, J. D. 1959. Dr. Louise Pearce. *Nature* **184** (August 22, 1959): 588–589.

Oakes, Elizabeth, ed. 2002. Pearce, Louise (1885–1959). In *International Encyclopedia of Women Scientists*. New York: Facts on File. 280–281.

Scholer, Anne-Marie. 1997. Louise Pearce (1885–1959). In *Women in the Biological Sciences: A Biobibliographic Sourcebook*. Edited by Louise S. Grinstein, Carol A. Biermann, and Rose K. Rose. Westport CT: Greenwood. 384–390.

12

ELIZABETH "LEE" HAZEN
(1885–1975)

Discoverer of Medically Useful Antifungal Antibiotics

Fungal infections can cause terrible diseases in humans and affect millions of people worldwide. Before 1950, there were no effective drugs to deal with such infections. Fungi are ubiquitous in nature and are omnipresent in soils and on plants of all kinds. They are so pervasive, it is likely that most people have been exposed to one or more pathogenic fungi at some point in their lives. Many of those exposed have developed one or more mycoses (fungal infections) but have not been aware of it because their natural defenses produced antibodies to ward off the microorganisms and provided a degree of immunity against further infection. Others whose defenses were not able to repel one of the many pathogenic fungi contracted one of the milder forms of the disease, like athlete's foot or ringworm. The most prevalent fungal disease usually experienced by age group 30–65 is acne (caused by *Propionibacterium acnes*).

Once the pathogenic fungi have gone out of control and enter the lymphatic system of the body, they disseminate, spreading to other parts of the body and producing infections that are all but impossible to arrest. Fungal disease may cause nonspecific symptoms of mild upper respiratory infection such as low-grade fever and cough or chills, sweating, and headaches. Further probing may reveal symptoms of pneumonia, tuberculosis, meningitis, rheumatoid arthritis, brain tumors or other afflictions. Unless the physician directs (and the laboratory performs) the highly specialized and time-consuming tests for pathogenic fungi the possible cause of the disease may not be found.

In 1950 Dr. Elizabeth Lee Hazen, an American scientist, along with Dr. Rachel Brown (1898–1980), discovered nystatin, an antifungal antibiotic, which provides an effective and safe treatment of human disease. Dr. Hazen led the search at the Albany laboratory for the New York State Health Department. She studied antibiotics useful in the control of fungal disease. She faced the same problems as Alexander Fleming (1881–1955), the discoverer of penicillin, namely how to extract and chemically define an active substance. She met Rachel Brown, an exceptionally talented, persevering organic chemist who was familiar with extraction of active ingredients from bacterial cultures. This collaboration resulted in finding the active principle in Hazen's strepto-mycete cultures and provided the evidence that it was highly active against a number of important fungi and only slightly toxic in experimental animals. They first called their agent "fungicidine" but renamed it "nystatin" after "New York State." The Brown-Hazen discovery of nystatin has proven to be the most effective agent against candida and aspergillus infections in the intes-tines, the vaginal tracts, the skin, and the mouth. If applied locally or taken orally, nystatin can help rid mucous membranes and other body surfaces of this disease.

Elizabeth Lee Hazen's career is a good example for us. She was a pioneer medical mycologist and also a good example of a pioneer woman scientist. In the 1940s, Hazen discovered that training in diagnosis of fungal disease — the mycoses — was meager or non-existent. Diagnostic trials were primitive as were the available tools, and specific antifungal drugs did not exist. In spite of the difficulties, Lee Hazen was determined to explore the new frontier, regardless of repeated gender discrimination.

Before Dr. Hazen began to study medical mycology there were several other microbiologists in pursuit of cures of fungal diseases. However, she was the first to accomplish that goal and met the growing need to combat fungal infections by following a deeply held belief "to develop the practical side of the sciences without sacrificing complete and accurate knowledge of princi-ples," a motto she lived by throughout her life.

Elizabeth Lee Hazen was born on August 24, 1885, in Rich, Coahoma County, Mississippi, a small farming community a few miles east of the Mis-sissippi River and some sixty miles south of Memphis, Tennessee. Her given first name was Lee. Her father was William Edgar Hazen and her mother was Maggie Harper. Lee was the second daughter of the family. She had a younger brother who died at a very young age. Both parents died before Lee was four years old. Lee and her sister were raised by their uncle and aunt, Robert Henry "Lep" Harper and Laura Crawford Hazen. They lived in the county in which the Hazen family had been established before the Civil War. Lee's grandfa-ther, Munson Hazen, a native of Vermont, had chosen to settle at nearby Friar's Point. When he was seventeen years old he purchased a 320 acre farm called "The Hazen Place" for less than fifty cents an acre. He later passed his land to Lee's parents when she was born. Lee was brought up by her uncle and aunt in a Baptist religious environment and attended church quite regularly. Interest in the Baptist religion continued throughout Lee's col-lege years. The Lula School that Lee attended in 1891 was an ungraded, one-room, one-teacher public school with about fifty students ranging from pre-school to high school age. Her academic record was outstanding and her teachers were supportive of Lee's ambition to excel.

Lee was an avid reader and spent many hours at the home library concentrating on history and biography, a preference she changed later when she entered science classes. (Conway Dickey, a cousin, donated Lee's library to the Mississippi University for Women after her death in 1975. He reported that there was not a single novel in the collection.) Despite her bookish attitude, she had a sparkling sense of humor and was very outspoken, not like the stereotype "bookworm." Clara Hazen, her "sister-cousin," recalled the valedictory address Lee gave in 1904 about Lucius Quinctius Cincinnatus Lamar, a revered Mississippi statesman who served as a U.S. representative, a senator, the secretary of the interior and an associate justice of the United States Supreme Court. Clara believed Lucius inspired Lee to set high goals for her life.

Upon completion of high school, Hazen received private tutoring sessions in Memphis. In 1905, she enrolled in the Mississippi Industrial Institute and College in Columbus (later Mississippi University for Women), where tuition was free and room and board cost as little as ten dollars per month. She decided to explore science with the most practical ends — the alleviation of human suffering. Her interest in science blossomed, in particular physiology, botany, zoology, physics, plant physiology and anatomy. She was an outstanding student and was one of thirty-five graduating from the college on May 27, 1910. She was also an active participant in extracurricular activities. It was noted in the graduating yearbook that she had been secretary and treasurer of the Baptist Missionary Society and assistant business manager of the campus newspaper, the *Spectators*; she was also a member of the cast of an all-girl theatrical production, "Men and Maids from Gay Paris." Her picture depicted a sweet, handsome young woman, immaculately dressed and with a serious look that typified her deeply held determination.

With her degree in hand, Hazen moved to Jackson, Mississippi, where she taught physics and biology at Central High School for six years. During that period, she attended summer sessions at the University of Tennessee, where she studied biology. She also attended the University of Virginia, where she took lecture and laboratory classes. In 1916 she entered Columbia University to continue her studies and received a master's degree in biology in 1917. During her enrollment at Columbia's College of Physicians and Surgeons, she offered her services to the U.S. War Department during World War I. By this time she had received the nickname "Elizabeth" from her new friends and associates and she continued to use that name. While in the Army, she worked as a technician in diagnostic laboratories in Camp Sheridan, Alabama, from 1918 to 1919, and in Camp Mills, New York, in 1919. The position gave her a lot of practical experience. She became assistant director of the Clinical and Bacteriological Laboratory of Cook Hospital in Fairmont, Virginia, where she remained until 1923.

In the fall of 1923 Hazen decided to go back to Columbia University for further graduate work in organic chemistry and to continue her study and research in the Department of Bacteriology and Immunology at the College of Physicians and Surgeons. On one of her research projects she wrote a report entitled "Unsuccessful Attempts to Cure or Prevent Tuberculosis in Guinea Pigs with Dreyer's Defatted Antigen." Her thesis was "General and Local Immunity to Ricin," which contained a list of fifty-nine references to the previous work along with accurate summaries of the earlier findings by microbiologists. In 1927 she published this article and received her Ph.D. in microbiology. She continued her research at Columbia until 1928, when she was appointed resident bacteriologist at the college-affiliated Presbyterian Hospital. She left that post to become a member of the teaching staff in the Department of Bacteriology and Immunology at the College of Physicians and Surgeons. This move allowed her to interact with many eager students.

Possibly a major turning point in her career came in 1931 when Augustus Wadsworth put her in charge of the Bacterial Diagnosis Laboratory in Albany, New York. This position was much to her liking and her performance led to increasing responsibilities, such as direct supervision of a large number of technicians, who were engaged in the examination of pathological specimens for the diagnosis of infectious diseases such as diphtheria, septic sore throat, typhoid fever, tuberculosis, gonorrhea, spinal meningitis and bacillary and amoebic dysentery. In addition, she supervised the work of the serum diagnosis department in which the test for syphilis was performed on thousands of blood and spinal fluid specimens. She also traced an outbreak of anthrax, a fatal disease in animals that is transmissible to men. She pinpointed sources of tularemia and also reported the first case in the United States of *Clostridium botulinum* Type E, a cause of poisoning from improperly preserved canned food. She also collaborated with Dr. Ruth Gilbert, the assistant director of the Diagnostic Laboratories of the Division of Laboratories and Research, and took pioneering studies of moniliasis (candidiasis). In spite of her strenuous schedule, she found time to attend lectures in organic chemistry and to study mycology in the Department of Dermatology. She studied in the Mycology Laboratory, which was established by Drs. J. Gardner Hopkins and Rhoda W. Benham (1894–1957). Dr. Benham was an authority on pathogenic fungi and under her supervision, Hazen collected and examined specimens taken from patients. Hazen also took cultures at the bed-side of patients and took them to the laboratory for further observation and identification of fungal agents. Elizabeth treasured every positive specimen, slide or culture, carefully preserving them all, not only for her own use, but — with Dr. Benham's encouragement — for the purpose of bringing them to her own laboratory, thus bringing mycological manna as well as gospel to her dis-ciples and associates at the Division of Laboratories and Research.

With the assistance of illustrator Frank C. Reed of the Division of Lab-oratories and Research, Elizabeth built a teaching collection of fungal cul-tures and slides in the Central Laboratory, which became a state-approved laboratory where special facilities had been made available to the physicians of the state for identification of fungi and related microorganisms. This col-lection served as a valuable teaching tool and later became a basis of her first book published in 1955, *Laboratory Diagnosis of Pathogenic Fungi Simplified*, a standard reference in the field. The second edition was published in 1960 and the third edition, co-authored with Morris A. Gordon, was published in 1970.

Dr. Hazen's strong desire to learn was not limited to diagnostic mycol-ogy. She undertook an independent investigation on *Microsporum audouinii*, which causes severe itching and loss of hair in school-aged children. She stud-ied the nutritional requirement of *M. audouinii* and worked to understand why macrospore production was induced when the fungus was grown together with *Bacillus weidmaniensis*. She published many papers on this subject. Her published works on mycological infections began to reveal her future direc-tion of work. She repeatedly stated in her published papers that the most promising antifungal preparations had no widespread application because of toxicity or other undesirable pharmacologic properties. She concluded, "Con-sequently, no antibiotic agent approaching the efficacy of penicillin and strep-tomycin against bacterial infections is available in fungal infections either of the superficial or the deep-seated type."

In 1948 Dr. Gilbert Dalldorf (b. 1900) became the director of the Divi-sion of the Laboratories and introduced Dr. Hazen to a collaborator, Dr. Rachel Brown of the Central Laboratory, who was a highly skilled chemist. With Dr. Dalldorf's strong endorsement and close collaboration with Dr. Brown, Dr. Hazen began intensive investigative screenings of soil samples in the search for microorganisms active against pathogenic fungi. She would eagerly open each new soil sample arriving at the branch laboratory, carefully labeling the place of origin and name of donor. A tiny amount of each sam-ple was mixed with sterile saline solution and seeded on a nutrient agar base until any actinomycetes had grown to the stage of visibility. These isolated cultures were then grown in liquid nutrient broth, plated in mason jars, labeled and shipped to Dr. Brown in Albany. Brown would extract active antibiotic ingredients from these mycotic cultures. Each mason jar received by Dr. Brown contained a whole culture, either static (a mixture of broth and a matted growth called the pellicle) or shaken (a suspension of the growth in the broth). Her first job was to determine the location of the active antifungal substance. Was it in the pellicle, the broth, or both? Hazen then tested whether the extractions from the fungi would stop fungal growth by inoculation of two pathogenic fungi in the laboratory. After preliminary tests, she mainly focused her research on the antifungal substances produced from just two of several actinomycetes collected. "No. 42705" proved to have good antifungal properties but was toxic to mice. "No. 48240" yielded two antifungal substances which Hazen was able to extract and separate. One extraction proved to be active against *Candida neoformans.* The other, extracted from the pellicle, showed considerable activity against both *C. albicans* and *C. neoformans.* As she obtained purer materials, those that showed the greatest potency against the test fungi were used by Hazen against actual fungal diseases induced by these pathogenic fungi in laboratory animals — mice and rabbits in this case. The animal experiments would show whether the antifungal activity seen in the laboratory was protective in living creatures and whether the substances were toxic in test animals and in humans. "No 48240" was given the name nystatin. Hazen established that the actinomycete from which nystatin was derived was a previously undiscovered microorganism called *Streptomyces noursei.* The organism was named after a friend, William B. Nourse, who had a farm near Warrenton, Virginia, from which a soil sample was taken that yielded the nystatin-producing actinomycetes. The samples Hazen tested were from compost, peat and manure as well as from various forest, field, and garden soil.

In the spring of 1951, the U.S. Patent Office issued a patent on nystatin to Drs. Hazen and Brown. They signed an agreement to allow Squibb Institute to manufacture and sell nystatin in the form of an antibiotic. In August 1954, the Food and Drug Administration approved the sale of nystatin tablets in oral dosage form as the first broadly effective antifungal antibiotic available to the medical profession. It was recommended for the prevention and treatment of intestinal moniliasis or candidiasis. In June 1957, nystatin was placed on the market with the patent commission's permission. Nystatin was effective against candida infections of the mouth and skin and intestinal as well as vaginal surfaces. Squibb eventually produced nystatin in various forms such as oral tablets and suspensions, creams, ointments, topical powders and vaginal tablets. When their patents expired in 1974, over thirteen million dollars had been generated. Half of the royalties were placed in the Brown-Hazen Fund, to be used to support research and training in the medical-biological sciences, to provide aid to women scientists in academic institutions and to add grant programs to continue the fight against fungal diseases. Furthermore, this fund also provided the American Type Culture in Rockville, Maryland, to collect, preserve, and distribute to the scientific community reference cultures of microorganisms, viruses, and animal and human cell lines.

Hazen's life was not disturbed by the discovery and the money generated. She continued her work vigorously. In 1954, the New York State branch laboratory was disbanded, but Dr. Hazen continued her research and diagnostic screening at the Central Laboratory in Albany. In 1958, Hazen accepted an associate professorship at Albany Medical College, where she retired in 1960. She then became a full-time guest investigator in the Columbia University Mycology Laboratory. In 1973 Hazen visited her ailing sister in Seattle, Washington. However, she was also ill, having suffered for many years from ulcers, and was unable to return to New York. She remained at the nursing home where her sister was. Two years later, on June 24, 1975, she died of acute cardiac arrhythmia at the age of 90.

Dr. Hazen received many awards in her later years. In 1955 she shared with Dr. Brown the Squibb Award in Chemotherapy. In 1968, she received a Distinguished Service Award from the New York State Department of Health. In 1975, a month before her death, Hazen and Brown were the first women to receive the Chemical Pioneer Award of the American Institute of Chemists.

Dr. Hazen came from a poor family. On her journey she had met considerable obstacles and endured personal sacrifice. She never married. She never presented a paper. She always avoided reporters and photographers in public. She was warm, outgoing and opinionated about matters of science and politics, and she was especially concerned about women's status in society. She was an extremely hard worker; her passion was her work.

*　*　*

Dr. Hazen's contributions were numerous. Her book *Laboratory Diagnosis of Pathogenic Fungi Simplified* was well received and gave impetus to a big advance in the basic science of medical mycology. Her discovery of antifungal antibiotics benefits humans immensely.

Dr. Hazen should be specially commended for her undying determination, perseverance, and patience in the microbiological and medical field. The cures she found for fungal diseases are still being administered worldwide.

Her work also reveals the need for scientists to be alert to fields other than their own immediate interests.

Dr. Hazen lived in an environment of gender discrimination, and undoubtedly she encountered problems because of her gender. However, her love for human beings and her hard-working attitude overcame much. Elizabeth Hazen's is a life to remember.

Further Reading

Bacon, W. S. 1976. Elizabeth Lee Hazen, 1888–1975. *Mycologia* (September/October): 961–969. (With the permission of SIM News, this article was reproduced from SIM News 49, 225–229, 1999.)

Baldwin, Richard S., and Gilbert Dalldorf. 1981. *The Fungus Fighters*. Ithaca NY: Cornell University Press.

Dixon, F. J., and Henry G. Kunkel. 1968. *Advances in Immunology* 9.

Rossiter, Margaret W. 1974. Women scientists in America before 1920. *American Scientists* (May–June): 312–323.

13

SARA ELIZABETH BRANHAM
(1888–1962)

Pioneer in Meningitis Studies

*If we look back carefully enough, with binoculars as it were, we may begin
to have some idea what went into the building of ancient structures, to appreciate the effort expended with primitive tools, to understand what went wrong
with the structures left unfinished, and to complete the work with new tools.—*
Sara Elizabeth Branham (1888–1962)

Dr. Sara Elizabeth Branham studied meningitis and contributed to the
advance in perfection and standardization of the anti-meningococcal antiserum. She also was the first to demonstrate that sulfa drugs were effective
against the infections caused by meningococci as well as against the dreaded
sequellae following these infections. Meningitis is an inflammation of the
meninges, the three protective membranes that cover the brain and spinal
cord. Meningitis can occur where there is an infection near the brain or spinal
cord, such as a respiratory infection in the sinus, the mastoids, or the cavi-
ties around the ear. Disease-causing organisms can travel to the meninges
through the bloodstream. The infected patients usually feel a severe headache
and neck stiffness followed by fever, vomiting, a rash, then convulsions leading to loss of consciousness.

Meningitis was one of the most dreaded diseases before sulfa drugs
became available in the early 1940s. Fatalities resulting from meningitis were
high among the young, and those who survived were at risk of severe after-
effects such as deafness, blindness, and mental retardation. Disastrous meningitis epidemics often occurred in army camps.

Today, bacterial meningitis is curable if treated promptly with antibiotics administered intravenously. Vaccines are available and a vaccine against
Haemophilus influenzae type b (Hib) is very effective. Dr. Branham's work
paved the way for much of the medical science that protects us against meningitis today.

Sara Elizabeth Branham was born July 25, 1888, in Oxford, Georgia. She came from a highly educated family. Her mother and grandmother were both graduates of Wesleyan College in Macon, Georgia, and both of her grandfathers had taught at Wesleyan and spent most of their lives teaching at Emory at Oxford. It was told that she was interested in biology from the time she was only three years old. She attended Palmer Institute in Georgia and graduated in 1904. She then attended Wesleyan College and obtained her A.B. degree in biology in 1907. After that, she taught science at girls' schools in Sparta, Decatur, and Atlanta for about 10 years. She developed a consuming interest in medical research, and her desire for learning was very strong; therefore, in 1917 she went to the University of Colorado in Boulder as an assistant in bacteriology, and in 1919, she obtained a second A.B. degree majoring in zoology and chemistry. Because of the shortage of manpower in World War I, she was given an opportunity to teach bacteriology at the University of Colorado Medical School. This opened doors for her future academic pursuits.

In 1920 she went to the University of Chicago and received an M.S. degree in bacteriology the same year. Three years later she obtained a Ph.D. in bacteriology. When she received her Ph.D., she returned briefly to the University of Colorado, Boulder, as an instructor. Having received a postdoctoral fellowship from the Douglas Smith Foundation for Medical Research, she resumed her studies at the University of Chicago in the fall of that year. In 1927, before completing her medical studies, she was appointed associate at the University of Rochester School of Medicine, New York, working with 'Dr. Stanhope Bayne-Jones (1888–1970). When she had been in Rochester only a few months, she was called to the Hygienic Laboratory of the United States Public Health Service (now called the National Institutes of Health, NIH) to do research on meningitis. Dr. Branham eagerly accepted the position as a bacteriologist and worked at NIH for thirty years until her retirement in 1958. During her tenure at NIH, she took a leave of absence in 1932 to complete requirements for the M.D. degree, which she received in 1934. While at NIH until 1952, Dr. Branham was a lecturer in preventive medicine at George Washington University, Washington, D.C. From 1959 to 1962, she was a visiting biologist of the American Institute for Biological Sciences.

While in Chicago, Dr. Branham worked for Dr. Edwin O. Jordan (1866–1936) on the project of isolating influenza viruses. She did not succeed because the state of art of virology was not ready for cultivation of viruses. Instead, she turned her efforts to the study of *Bacterium enteritidis* (now called *Salmonella enteritidis*). She demonstrated the toxicity and antigenic properties of the culture filtrate, which contains the soluble antigens and a specific carbohydrate that reacted with specific antisera. Dr. Branham published a paper in 1928 coauthored by L. Robey and L. A. Day. The title of her paper was "A Poison Produced by *Bacterium enteritidis* and *Bacterium aertrycke* Which Is Active in Mice When Given by Mouth." She clearly demonstrated the poison produced by these microorganisms, which were the most commonly encountered members of the paratyphoid group that cause food poisoning.

A serious epidemic of cerebrospinal meningitis occurred in China and reached California in 1927 when Dr. Branham was called to work at NIH. The meningitis was caused by a new strain of *Neisseria meningitidis* (commonly called meningococcus). This organism was difficult to work with in the laboratory since to remain viable it required subculture every second day to keep the culture alive. The standard antiserum that had been used since 1904 was no longer effective. In 1909 Dr. Louise Pearce (1885–1959) of the Rockefeller Institute traveled to France to obtain the typed meningococcus cultures from Dr. Charles Dopter (b.1873). She transferred the cultures every second day to keep the culture alive. The standard antiserum had been prepared from these strains of meningococcus. Specific antiserum was the only known therapy during the epidemic years of World War I. The epidemic of meningitis and associated research stopped when the war ended. By 1928 serum therapy appeared to be completely ineffective because only a few laboratories maintained the culture, and the old stock culture slowly lost the antigenicity with each transfer. Dr. Branham had to make a special trip to England, where Drs. M. H. Gordon and E. D. G. Murray had retained their type strain of *N. meningitidis* in dried conditions. Dr. Branham prepared monovalent serum for typing each live organism that was sent to her at the Hygienic Laboratory. All of the new strains she collected still had to be transferred every second day.

The knowledge related to meningitis increased rapidly. Soon it was found that Gordon and Murray's type I and type III strains were not separable except by agglutinin absorption and that their capsular polysaccharides were identical. Therefore, these strains were placed in Group 1. Dr. Branham discovered that more than 95 percent of the strains causing epidemics belonged to Group 1; hence, this group was known as the epidemic group and subsequently designated Group A. Later it was demonstrated that most chronic carriers have Group B organisms, and a Group C was described later.

Using experimentally infected animals such as guinea pigs and mice, Dr. Branham demonstrated clearly that the virulence of the pathogen carried by patients determined the occurrence of the epidemic of meningitis. She also found that the differences in virulence in the S (smooth) and R (rough) colonies correlated with antigenic differences. It was also demonstrated that the agglutination tests carried at 37° C were much more specific than those at 55° C overnight incubation. She continued to improve the agglutination method, which could be used in direct typing of organisms isolated from cerebral fluids of patients. Dr. Branham hired Dr. Margaret Pittman (1901–1995), one of her former students at the University of Chicago. Together they worked out a standard method for the titration of antiserum that was used for therapy of meningococcus infections.

As mentioned before, antiserum was the only treatment for meningitis before the availability of sulfa drugs. Dr. Branham was the first to demonstrate that sulfa drugs were effective against infection caused by meningococcus. Meningococci were later shown to be sensitive to penicillin and some other broad spectrum antibiotics, but they quickly acquired resistance to streptomycin and even developed dependency on it. Sulfadiazine became the drug of choice for treatment of the meningitis infections.

Dr. Branham also studied the toxins produced by *Shigella dysenteriae*, a pathogen causing serious diarrhea called bacterial dysentery. The toxin was called Shiga toxin. She irradiated toxin to produce toxoids and discovered that antiserum (antitoxin) would be protective to the experimental animals if given at the early stage of infection. However, Shiga antitoxin was later found to be a poor therapeutic agent because the Shiga toxin had such a marked affinity for the nervous system that its effects were not reversed by antitoxins. Using monkeys as experimental animals, Dr. Branham illustrated that subcutaneous or intravenous injections of toxin produced by *S. dysenteriae* would produce characteristic clinical symptoms. She also found that Shiga toxin was perfectly innocuous when in contact with normal intestinal mucosa of monkeys, although toxin was fatal when given parenterally. She demonstrated that the toxin was detoxified before absorption from the intestinal pouch.

In addition, Dr. Branham studied the antigenicity of *Shigella sonnei* in relation to the culture phase of this organism. She showed that phase II cultures were remarkably antigenic and virulent to mice. She also studied the toxin produced by *Cornyebacterium diphtheriae,* and she demonstrated an additional component in the antigen from these bacterial cultures. Other aspects of her research involved the effect of cortisone and adrenocorticotrophic hormone (ACTH) on adrenals in experimental diphtheria, shigella, and meningococcus intoxications. No effect of these hormones on the outcome of the experimental infection in guinea pigs was found.

Dr. Branham was well known and recognized for her work on meningitis. A chapter on the chemistry of antigens written by Branham was included in *Newer Knowledge of Bacteriology and Immunology* (1928). She also contributed a chapter on laboratory diagnosis of meningococcus meningitis and identification of the meningococcus to *Yearbook Supplement of the American*

Journal of Public Health in 1935. In 1941 she contributed a similar chapter in *Recommended Procedures and Reagents* of the American Public Health Association, first edition, and in 1945 the second edition. In the third edition of the American Public Health Association, she wrote a chapter entitled "The Meningitis." A similarly broad review of bacterial meningitis also appeared in 1963, fourth edition. Dr. Branham was also one of the authors of the tenth edition of *Practical Bacteriology, Hematology and Parasitology*, which was a standard text for many years.

In addition, Dr. Branham contributed greatly to the taxonomy of Neisseria. With the collaboration of Dr. E. G. D. Murray, she prepared a section on the genus Neisseria for *Bergey's Manual of Determinative Bacteriology* in 1948 and again in 1957. She also prepared a section on reference strains for the serological groups of meningococcus that appeared in the *International Bulletin of Bacterial Nomenclature and Taxonomy*. She was appointed to the International Subcommittee of the Family of Neisseriaceae Nomenclature, in which she served as secretary for several years. She was influential in the development of the classification scheme of Neisseria. In recognition of Dr. Branham's outstanding contributions to knowledge of the Neisseria, the genus Branhamella was created in her honor in 1974 for the non-pathogen, formerly designated *Neisseria catarrhalis*, which she had differentiated from the pathogenic *N. meningitidis* and *N. gonorrheae*.

Dr. Branham was bestowed with numerous honors. She received the Howard Taylor Ricketts Prize for research in pathology in 1924. She was awarded an honorary Doctor of Science degree in 1937 from the University of Colorado. She was the recipient of the Alumni Award for outstanding achievement from Wesleyan College in 1950. The Distinguished Service Award from the University of Chicago Alumnae was given to her in 1952; and she was named Woman of the Year by the American Medical Women's Association in 1959. Additionally, she was listed in *Who's Who in America* in 1945.

Dr. Branham had been active in many scientific societies. She was president of the Tungsten Chapter of Iota Sigma Pi (Women Chemists Association) in 1918–1919. She was a member of the Society of American Bacteriologists (now called American Society for Microbiology) and served as president of the Washington Branch, 1937–1938, and councilor for many years. She chaired the Laboratory Section of the American Public Health Association 1946–1947 and was a councilor 1947–1952. Dr. Branham was elected president of the D.C. Chapter of Sigma Xi for 1953–1955. She attended many scientific meetings; notably she was an official delegate to the first and second International Congress for Microbiology in Paris, 1930, and London, 1936, respectively. She prepared recorded lectures on "Meningococcus Meningitis" for distribution to the University of Chungking, China, 1950.

Dr. Branham lived a happy life. She was a petite woman of grace and charm with zest for life. She came from a warm and supportive family. She prepared herself with good education and entered an inspiring field of bio-medical research. Her penchant for meticulous details in research led to a great contribution to science and humanity. At home, she maintained a beautiful garden and enjoyed the serenity of home life. She loved literature. Her lectures were often enlivened with literary references from her classical background in the arts. Dr. Branham often emphasized that we should look back carefully at everything we had done, because from that perspective we could understand both successes and failures and perhaps use the understanding to achieve new advances. In 1945, at the age of 57, Dr. Branham married Philip S. Mathews, a retired businessman. She enjoyed a brief (only four years) but happy life with him. Mr. Mathews died in 1949, and she never married again. On November 16, 1962, at age 74, Dr. Branham died suddenly from a heart attack. She was buried in her family plot in Oxford, Georgia.

*   *   *

Dr. Branham came from a family ahead of its time in its belief in higher education for women, and Dr. Branham fulfilled that noble belief. Her life and work are monumental to the achievement of women in medicine and public health. She set a good example for all of us to follow. She researched a terrible disease and made a marvelous contribution to mankind. She surely helped us to live better.

14

REBECCA CRAIGHILL LANCEFIELD
(1895–1981)

Researcher of Streptococci Classification and Infections

Rebecca Craighill Lancefield developed an immunological system for the classification of streptococci, which was later called the Lancefield system. The Lancefield system has contributed greatly to the medical understanding of streptococcal diseases including sore throat, puerperal sepsis, endocarditis, pericarditis, rheumatic fever, scarlet fever, pneumonia, and kidney infections. Dr. R.G. Lancefield's laboratory at the Rockefeller Institute for Medical Research (now Rockefeller University) has been called "the Scotland Yard of streptococcal mysteries." Her work is referred to in many microbiological textbooks today.

Rebecca Price Craighill was born on January 5, 1895, in Fort Wadsworth on Staten Island in New York. Her father was William Edward Craighill. The Craighill family came from Virginia, where they settled in the early 1800s. Mr. William E. Craighill graduated from West Point and was an army officer in the Army Corps of Engineers. Rebecca's mother was Mary Montagu Byram, a direct descendent of Lady Mary Wortley Montagu (1689–1762), who promoted smallpox immunization in the early 18th century in England. Mary's brother was a West Point classmate of William E. Craighill. Through this association, Mary and William became acquainted and then married.

Rebecca received a good education. In 1912 she entered Wellesley College, majoring in English and French initially, later changing to zoology. She obtained her bachelor's degree in 1916. After graduation, she accepted a job teaching physical geography in a girls' boarding school (Hopkins Hall) in Burlington, Vermont. She was able to save $200 from her annual salary of $500 and was offered a scholarship to attend graduate school at Teacher's College of Columbia University in New York.

Rebecca was interested in bacteriology; however, she could not study the subject at the Teacher's College. Thus, she pursued her graduate work in bacteriology at the College of Physicians and Surgeons of Columbia University under the supervision of the world renowned bacteriologist Dr. Hans Zinsser (1878–1940). She earned a master's degree in 1918 and in the same year married Donald Lancefield, who was her classmate in the drosophila genetics course taught by Nobel Prize laureate Dr. T. H. Morgan (1866–1945).

During World War I, Donald Lancefield was called into military service. At the beginning of his service, while still a private, he was stationed with the Sanitary Corps Unit at the Rockefeller Institute for Medical Research, where he attended a special course conducted in part by Dr. Oswald T. Avery (1877–1955) and Dr. Aphonse R. Dochez (1882–1964). Rebecca Lancefield, having just finished her master's degree, applied to the Rockefeller Institute for a research position. She started as a technician at the Rockefeller Hospital working in the laboratory of Drs. Oswald Avery and Aphonse Dochez. The young newlyweds were thus working at the Rockefeller Institute at that time.

Drs. Avery and Dochez were well known for their work on pneumococci, responsible for pneumonia and other diseases. Much of their work was done during World War I when epidemics of pneumonia were common. There was a big outbreak of pneumonia in a military camp in Texas. Drs. Avery and Dochez's research project at Rockefeller Institute was to determine if a distinctive type of pneumococcus could be isolated from soldiers in the Texas military camp. Rebecca employed the same serological techniques that Avery had used to distinguish types of pneumococci. In 1919 she published a paper in the *Journal of Experimental Medicine* titled "Studies on the Biology of Streptococcus. 1. antigenic relationships between strains of *Streptococcus haemolyticus*," which described four types of streptococci. This work was the beginning of her career as an expert of streptococcal classification.

For three months, during the summer of 1919, both Rebecca and her husband worked at the Marine Biological Laboratory in Woods Hole, Massachusetts. After returning to New York, Rebecca was a research assistant for Dr. C. W. Metz (1889–1975) in his genetic laboratory at Columbia. She did cytological and genetic studies of *Drosophila willistoni* and other species. She published three papers as a result of this work.

In 1921 Rebecca went to Oregon, which was the home state of her husband, who finished his doctoral requirements and was offered a position at the University of Oregon. Rebecca found a position teaching bacteriology at the same university. The following year, both of them returned to New York. Dr. Donald Lancefield joined the Columbia University faculty in Dr. Morgan's department. He remained on the faculty for many years until he became the chairman of the department of zoology at Queens College in New York. Rebecca enrolled in the Ph.D. program at Columbia University and did research on rheumatic fever at the Rockefeller Institute.

Rebecca worked in the laboratory of Dr. Homer Swift (1881–1953). At this time physicians suspected that rheumatic fever was caused by a streptococcus. But Dr. Swift and other scientists had not been able to isolate a specific organism from rheumatic fever patients, nor could they reproduce the disease in animals using cultures isolated from patients. Rebecca's research was to test many streptococci to see whether they could produce rheumatic fever in animals. She finally concluded that the alpha-hemolytic class of streptococci (also called green or viridans, i.e., *Streptococcus viridans*) was not the cause of rheumatic fever. These findings became the basis of her 1925 Ph.D. dissertation titled *The Immunological Relationships of* Streptococcus viridans *and Certain of Its Chemical Fractions*. This resulted in two papers published in the *Journal of Experimental Medicine*.

Dr. R. Lancefield's interest in rheumatic fever did not stop at this point. She thought that it was necessary to take a basic approach to study the potential pathogens. She began to recognize types among the disease-causing beta-hemolytic streptococci using the serological techniques developed by Avery. Her main tool was the precipitin test that involves mixing soluble type-specific antigens (usually the bacterial cells) with antisera (types of serum containing antibodies, generally IgG or IgM) to form large, interlocking molecular aggregates called lattices, which give a visible precipitate.

From the precipitin test, Dr. R. Lancefield discovered two surface antigens from these streptococci. One was a polysaccharide complex called C substance. This polysaccharide complex is a major component of the cell wall in all streptococci. Based on the different compositions of the polysaccharide complex, she further subdivided them into different groups designated by the letters *A* through *O*. The most common species causing human disease, *Streptococcus pyogenes*, were placed in group A. Within the group A streptococci, Dr. R. Lancefield found another important antigen, called M protein. The M protein is not identical in all streptococci. Based on differences in M protein composition, she subdivided group A streptococci into more than 60 different types.

About this time, Frederick Griffith (1879–1941) also did research in England on the classification of streptococci. Griffith's typing of streptococci was based on a slide agglutination method in which the bacteria in serum clump when a specific antibody is introduced. Lancefield and Griffith exchanged samples and information and verified each other's work. Unfortunately, Frederick Griffith was killed in 1941 during the bombing of London in World War II. Ultimately, Dr. R. Lancefield's system, based on the M protein types, was selected as the universal standard for classifying group A streptococci.

Lancefield found that M protein was responsible for the bacterial virulence and inhibited the white blood cells from engulfing the streptococci. This was different from the finding of Avery, who had discovered that virulence in the pneumococcus was due to a polysaccharide, not a protein. Further studies indicated that M protein is an important protein that elicits protective immune responses.

Lancefield continued to group streptococci obtained from different laboratories around the world into types. She painstakingly and thoroughly investigated the complexity and diversity of the different serotypes of these bacteria and established the classification system, which is still in use today.

Dr. R. Lancefield was also interested in the pathogenesis of streptococci. She demonstrated the connection between the bacteria constituents, primarily the M protein compositions, and the baffling nature of streptococcal diseases. She found that M protein is very type-specific and that the acquired immunity to one group A serotype could not protect against infections caused by other serotypes in group A. Later in the 1950s, Dr. R. Lancefield and Dr. Gertrude Perlmann purified the M protein and developed a good method for typing it. In addition to the M protein of the group A streptococci, she also characterized other group A protein antigens, which were designated T and R. She also worked on group B streptococci. She clarified the role of their polysaccharide in virulence and demonstrated how protein antigens on their surface protected their infections. Her work greatly helped in fighting the high rate of births in which infants carried group B infections that resulted in meningitis. That was a serious public health problem during the 1970s and is still a problem today.

Additionally, she often followed the medical records of rheumatic fever patients. She found that once patients had acquired immunity to a serotype, their immunities could last up to thirty years. She demonstrated that high titers (or concentration of antibody) could persist in the absence of antigens. However, Lancefield stressed that someone could suffer recurrent attacks of rheumatic fever because each one was caused by a different serotype.

During World War II, Dr. R. Lancefield served in the Army and performed special duties on the Streptococcal Diseases Commission of the Armed Forces Epidemiological Board. She identified strains from bacterial infections and provided antisera for epidemics of scarlet and rheumatic fevers in military camps. This commission was called the "Strep Club" and after the war ended, her colleagues created the Lancefield Society in 1977. The Lancefield Society has been responsible for regular annual international conferences on advances in streptococcal research.

Dr. R. Lancefield worked in the Rockefeller Institute almost all of her life. She became an associate member in 1946 and a full member and professor in 1958. In 1965 she retired but held emeritus professor status and continued to work in the laboratory until November 1980, when she broke her hip. She died of complications from the injury on March 3, 1981, at the age of eighty-six. Her husband Donald died the following August.

Dr. R. Lancefield worked in a field dominated by men, and she did not want any special recognition as a woman scientist. Most of her recognition came in the latter part of her life. She was elected president of the American Society for Microbiology (ASM) in 1943. In 1961 she was the first woman elected president of the American Association of Immunologists, and in 1970 she was one of few women elected to the National Academy of Sciences. Other honors included the T. Duckett Jones Memorial Award in 1960, the American Heart Association Award in 1964, the New York Academy of Medicine Medal in 1973, a Research Achievement Award for the *Journal of Medicine* in 1973, and honorary degrees from Rockefeller University in 1973 and Wellesley College in 1976. She was also awarded an Honorary Fellowship of the Royal College of Pathologists in 1976.

We know little of Dr. Rebecca Lancefield's childhood, but we are sure that she was an eager learner and was persistent to pursue her interest. She saved money from her first job as a teacher in a girls' boarding school in order to pursue graduate education. She found a way to study bacteriology, her field of interest, even though the school in which she enrolled did not teach the subject. She persistently focused on her interest and did diligently the work she considered significant. Ultimately, she made a great contrition both to science and to human health.

In addition to research, she enjoyed her family. She had one daughter and was fond of swimming and playing tennis with her family. Because her laboratories in Rockefeller Institute were not air conditioned, she would spend the summer season in Woods Hole, Massachusetts, with her family. She was a devoted worker maintaining a low profile, and she preferred not to go on lecture tours or attend scientific meetings. She continued to drive to Rockefeller Laboratory from her home in Douglaston, Long Island, to work even after her retirement.

*   *   *

As Joshua Lederberg (1925–) said, "Try hard to find out what you are good at, and what your passions are, and where the two converge, and build your life around that. Make deliberate choices, do not wait for things to happen." Dr. Rebecca Lancefield's life experience was a witness of the above statement. She found her interest and devoted herself to doing the best. She had a fulfilling life and also contributed greatly to human society.

Although the recognition of Dr. Rebecca Lancefield's contributions came in the later part of her life, she was one of the few who does not seem to have experienced gender discrimination.

Since rheumatic fever is still the leading cause of heart disease in the young in the developing world, there is still much to be learned about the disease. The legacy of the Lancefield system remains useful, and Dr. Rebecca Lancefield's name will always be remembered by microbiologists.

Further Reading

McCarty, M. 1987. Rebecca Craighill Lancefield. *Biographical Memoirs, National Academy of Sciences* 57: 226–246.
O'Hern, E. M. 1985. *Profiles of Pioneer Women Scientists.* New York: Acropolis. 69–78.
Schwarts, J. N. 1990. Mrs. L. *Research Profiles* (Summer): 1–6.
Wannamaker, L. 1981. Rebecca Craighill Lancefield. *American Society for Microbiology News* 47: 555–558.

15

GERTY THERESA RADNITZ CORI
(1896–1957)

Researcher in Sugar Metabolism and Glycogen Storage Disorders

This I believe, for a research worker the unforgotten moments of his life are those rare ones, which come after years of plodding work, when the veil over nature's secret seems suddenly to lift, and when what was dark and chaotic appears in a clear and beautiful light and pattern. —Gerty Cori (1896–1957)

Gerty Theresa Radnitz Cori was a biochemist who pioneered research on sugar metabolism and elucidated the mechanisms of cellular glycogen storage disorders. Her discoveries are included in fundamental biochemical textbooks today. Because exceptions help define the norm, her work helps us to understand not only the basic mechanisms of sugar metabolism but also the role of sugar metabolism in fighting diseases. She was the first woman to receive a Nobel Prize in Medicine or Physiology in 1947, along with her husband, Dr. Carl Ferdinand Cori (1896–1984), and Dr. Bernardo A. Houssay (1887–1971). Nobel Prizes were previously awarded to two other women: Marie Curie (1867–1934) in 1903 (Physics) and 1911 (Chemistry) and Irène Joliot-Curie (1897–1956) in 1935 (Chemistry).

Gerty Radnitz was born on August 15, 1896, in Prague, which was then a part of the Austro-Hungarian Empire (now the capital of the Czech Republic). Her father was Otto Radnitz, a manager of sugar refineries, and her mother was Martha Neustadt Radnitz. She was the first of three daughters; the other two sisters were Lotte and Hilda. The family was moderately wealthy, and the children grew up in a comfortable Prague apartment and had private tutors. At age ten, Gerty entered a lyceum for girls, which gave very little emphasis to science and mathematics but greatly stressed the development of cultural and social graces. At the age of 16, she was especially interested in chemistry and decided to study medicine. Even though she was ill prepared, her uncle Robert, a professor of pediatrics at Carl Ferdinand University, encouraged her.

In the summer of 1912, while vacationing in the Tyrol, she met a teacher from the *Tetschen Realgymnasium* who helped her in her study of Latin. Gerty took just one year to master the courses she needed to pass the special entrance examination called *Matura*, which tested the subjects of Latin, literature, history, mathematics, physics, and chemistry. This was a tough examination — as Gerty later said, "the hardest examination I was ever called upon to take." When World War I broke out in 1914, Gerty was admitted to Carl Ferdinand University. She was proud to be admitted to an institution with a longstanding heritage, for the university had been established in 1348. The university was divided into two branches, Czech and German, and Gerty chose the German branch.

Gerty met a fellow student, Carl Ferdinand Cori, during the first semester in an anatomy class at the university. She was a pretty, vivacious, brown-eyed girl with a mass of reddish-brown hair and a slender figure. Carl was a tall, shy, fair-haired, and blue-eyed handsome young man. They were the same age, and both loved sports such as mountain climbing in the Austrian Alps, swimming, skating, and tennis. It did not take long for them to fall in love with each other, but both were determined to get their medical degrees before they married. Also they were temporarily separated by the war as Carl served on the Alpine trails until the war ended, then transferred to the sanitary corps where he almost died of typhoid fever.

Together, they shared a common interest in scientific research. Gerty Radnitz and Carl Cori collaborated on several subjects, including a study of the complement of human serum — a group of serum proteins involved in white blood cell phagocytosis that plays a key role in immune responses by combining with antibodies. They coauthored research papers and established a lifelong collaboration. In 1920 both graduated from medical school.

Shortly after their graduation they moved to Vienna and married on August 5, 1920. It was a happy period in their lives, and since they were free from school, they could indulge in the sports they loved. One of their favorite activities was climbing glaciers.

After the devastating war ended in 1918, the new nation of Czechoslovakia needed medical doctors to revitalize healthcare. Soon, Carl Cori was offered a position at the University of Vienna, working half time at the Pharmacology Laboratory and half time in the Internal Medicine Department. He was appointed assistant in pharmacology at the University of Graz, Austria, the next year. From 1920 to 1922 Gerty Cori worked as an assistant at the Karolinen Children's Hospital in Vienna. While doing chemical work and research, she noticed that some of her young patients suffered from a disease called congenital myxedema (cretinism), which was induced by the severe dysfunction of the thyroid glands. Patients with congenital myxedema were characterized by swelling and thickening around the lips and mental deterioration. She published several papers on her studies of the thyroid and the spleen.

Despite the hard work of both Coris, life was not easy for them in the early 1920s. Europe was still in the midst of great social and economic unrest after World War I. There were food shortages in some regions, and Gerty suffered from malnutrition while working in Vienna. Due to the upheaval caused by the war, doing scientific research was extremely difficult because of poor funding and lack of supplies. The Coris saw little hope for their scientific future. They felt a strong urge to do scientific work in an environment free of strife. The Coris had experienced firsthand the conflicts, sorrows, and suffering of mankind at war, and it became their determination to make a contribution to the alleviation of these sufferings. Moving to the United States in order to be able to continue their medical research was one of their desires. In 1922 Carl Cori got a research position in biochemistry at the New York State Institute for the Study of Malignant Diseases in Buffalo (later called Roswell Park Memorial Institute). Gerty Cori joined him a few months later and was hired as an assistant pathologist at the same institute. She became an assistant biochemist in 1925.

The Coris never regretted their decision to migrate to the U.S.A. Years later, Gerty commented: "The high state of development of biochemical methods in the United States came as a revelation. The Institute offered good equipment and complete freedom in the choice of problems."

Gerty Cori was a persistent and diligent researcher. She followed her earlier observation on how the thyroid affects the body temperature. Their first publication in English was a report on the influence of thyroid extract on the growth and replication of the protozoan paramecium. However, since the couple was working in an institute that specialized in malignant diseases, they were pressured to investigate cancers. Nevertheless, they managed to explore other fields; their publications covered topics from the biological effects of X-rays to the effects of restricted diets on metabolism. However, their colleagues attacked their working together as a team. The director of the institute threatened to dismiss Gerty Cori if she continued her collaborative work on the metabolism of tumors with her husband. Their colleagues argued that collaboration would hurt Carl Cori's career as the low status of a woman researcher would tarnish the quality of research.

The Coris ignored their warnings and worked closely together. When

Gerty had some free time, she devoted it completely to the study of carbohydrate metabolism. Within a few years the Coris' work on how the body burns and stores sugars became known worldwide. They were at the cutting edge in the field of human sugar metabolism and, therefore, published a number of papers that changed medical perspectives.

Both became naturalized citizens of the United States in 1928. As their reputations grew, Carl Cori was offered the chair of the Department of Pharmacology at the Washington University School of Medicine, St. Louis, Missouri. Despite a university rule that two members of the same family could not be employed in the same department, Gerty Cori was given a token salary as a research fellow (1931–1938). Later she became a research associate in the Pharmacology Department (1938–1942). The couple continued working on sugar metabolism, and their laboratories became an international center for biochemical research. At the same time, they nurtured many promising students or visiting scientists including five future Nobel laureates: Christian de Duve (1917–), Arthur Kornberg (1918–), Luis F. Leloir (1906–1987), Severo Ochoa (1905–2000), and Earl Sutherland, Jr. (1915–1974). Also, many other distinguished scientists spent some time in their laboratories working with them on various subjects. Gerty Cori gave lectures occasionally and conducted seminars for staff as well as medical and graduate students. Although at first she was a little shy in giving lectures, feeling uncomfortable every time she faced a classroom, she became perfectly at ease after many years of experience. Her lectures sparkled with clarity and conciseness. Gerty Cori became an associate research professor of biological chemistry and pharmacology in 1942 and full professor in 1947, only after both Coris received their highest scientific honor, the Nobel Prize.

Before the Coris' discovery, medical scientists believed that glucose in blood was formed from another carbohydrate, glycogen, which was discovered by Claude Bernard (1813–1878). Glycogen is a natural polymer consisting of a large number of glucose molecules bonded together; it is stored in the liver and muscle. The belief was that glycogen could be broken down into glucose simply by hydrolysis, which did not require enzymes. By and large the glucose content of the blood is constant in a healthy person. When sugar intake is high, storage of glycogen in the liver increases, and when the blood glucose levels fall below normal, the glycogen of the liver is converted into glucose, which enters the bloodstream. Gerty and Carl Cori discovered that glycogen is broken down into glucose not by simple hydrolysis but by an enzyme called phosphorylase, and the product of phosphorylase is glucose-1-phosphate, not glucose. Glucose-1-phosphate was a new compound at the time, and it was sometimes termed the Cori ester. Further study unraveled more steps of the complex process of glucose metabolism. Glucose-1-phosphate is further converted to glucose-6-phosphate by another enzyme called phosphoglucomutase. Glucose-6-phosphate can be further metabolized into other products. Each step is mediated by one specific enzyme. This work opened up research on how carbohydrates are used, stored, and metabolized in the body. The Coris' work changed the way scientists thought about reactions in the human body and laid down the foundation for the understanding of the major metabolic pathway — glycolysis or the Embden-Meyerhof pathway.

After insulin was discovered in 1922 by Sir Frederick Grant Banting (1891–1941), Charles H. Best (1899–1978), and John James Rickard Macleod (1876–1935), the Coris immediately examined the role of this hormone on sugar metabolism. In 1924 Gerty and Carl compared sugar levels in the blood of both arteries and veins under the influence of insulin and found that in the absence of this hormone, the sugar level increased. At the same time they examined why tumors used large amounts of glucose in the tissues.

They also determined the rate of absorption of various sugars from the intestine and measured the level of several products of sugar metabolism, including lactic acid and glycogen. More importantly, they studied the effect of insulin on the metabolism of sugar in both muscles and liver. From these studies they proposed a cycle, now called the Cori cycle, to interpret the relationships between glucose, glycogen, and lactic acid. These relationships include how blood glucose becomes muscle glycogen, muscle glycogen becomes blood lactic acid, blood lactic acid becomes liver glycogen, and liver glycogen becomes blood glucose. The Coris' work generated much excitement among the biochemical research communities and elucidated many complex processes of carbohydrate metabolism. Both Gerty and Carl Cori's contributions to the understanding of carbohydrate metabolism are fundamental to modern biochemistry.

Gerty Cori never forgot her early interest in pediatric medicine. As she grew older, she returned her attention to a group of inherited childhood diseases known collectively as glycogen storage disorders. She studied the structure of the highly branched glycogens. Through studies of glycogen metabolism and properties of their metabolic enzymes, she found that the disorders of glycogen storage could be categorized into two groups: one involved too much glycogen, and the other was involved with abnormal glycogen. Both of these diseases originated from the dysfunction of enzymes that control the glycogen metabolism. This work also opened up a new field of study in which the understanding of the structure and function of enzymes could be critical in interpreting the origins of diseases. She also investigated the mechanisms of action of hormones produced by the pituitary glands.

Well-known biochemist Ernst Starling (b. 1905) said, "The physiology of today is the medicine of tomorrow." It would be hard to find a more fitting statement to describe the Coris' contribution to the understanding of sugar metabolism and diabetes.

Gerty Cori received numerous awards for her contribution to science. In addition to the Nobel Prize, she was a recipient of the Midwest Award from the American Chemical Society (1946), the Lasker Award of the American Public Health Association (1946), the Squibb Award in Endocrinology (1947), the St. Louis Award (1948), the Garvan Medal for women chemists of the American Chemical Society (1948), the Sugar Research Prize from the National Academy of Sciences (1950), and the Borden Award from the Association of Medical Colleges (1951).

She also received honorary doctorates from Boston University in 1948, Smith College in 1949, Yale University in 1951, Columbia University in 1954, and the University of Rochester in 1955. Gerty Cori was elected a member of the National Academy of Sciences in 1948. She was also an active member of many scientific societies including the American Philosophical Society, the American Society of Biological Chemists, the Harvey Society, the American Chemical Society, and the Sigma Xi Society.

In 1952 President Harry Truman appointed her to the science board of the National Science Foundation. She made many trips to Washington, D.C., despite her poor health.

In Missouri, Gerty and Carl lived in a pleasant but small house outside of the city. Their beautiful home was filled with flowers, art, books, and music. Gerty liked the music of Bach, Beethoven and Mozart. "I believe that in art and sciences are the glories of the human minds," she wrote. She also loved the paintings of Dürer, Rembrandt, and the Impressionists.

The Coris' lifestyle was simple and unostentatious. Gerty drove a war-weary 1941 Ford to work every day. She and her husband went to few parties and concerts, preferring the enjoyment of work and family. According to Dr. Mildred Cohn (b. 1913), Gerty was energetic, kind, and compassionate, while Carl was more aloof, easy-going, and had an excellent sense of humor. Gardening was a special hobby for both of them, and they worked as a team. Gerty took care of the flowers, and Carl tended the vegetables.

Edward Doisy (1893–1986), a Nobel laureate who discovered vitamin K, once said, "Genius the Coris have, there is no question about it. But their capacity for hard work has aided that genius to blossom and to benefit mankind. They are good Americans, excellent companions, the kind that fishermen like to take to the woods with them. They are swimmers as well and all-around outdoor people."

Gerty was climbing Snowmass Mountain in Colorado in the summer of 1947 when she first noticed the symptoms of myelofibrosis, a rare bone marrow disease. Although she had to receive numerous blood transfusions, she kept doing research. Her courage was astonishing. She did many brave things in her life. Enduring her illness was one, and having her first child, Thomas, at the age of 40 was another. During her last ten years she had to slow down her activities and put away her tennis racket, ice skates, and climbing equipment. But the more she weakened the more courage she showed. She continued to work in the laboratory, showing extra kindness to foreign students who felt lonely. She wrote, "Intellectual integrity, courage, and kindness are still the virtues I admire though with advancing years the emphasis has been slightly shifted, and kindness has seemed more important to me than in my youth." She died of complications of myelofibrosis on October 27, 1957, in St. Louis, Missouri. She was cremated, and her ashes rest in St. Louis.

Carl Cori later married Anne Fitzgerald Jones on August 23, 1960, and retired from Washington University in 1966. He then was visiting professor at the Harvard University School of Medicine and died on August 20, 1984, in Cambridge, Massachusetts.

Gerty and Carl Cori's son, Carl Thomas Cori, who was born in 1936 in St. Louis, Missouri, earned a Ph.D. degree and became a research chemist.

*   *   *

It is impossible to separate Gerty and Carl Cori's contributions. They collaborated intimately as a team, and together they were stronger than either of them would have been alone. They coauthored over two hundred research articles. They were equally creative and hard taskmasters; nonetheless, society in their time did not provide them with equal rewards. As in most professions, women were less valued and their work and views suspect. Both were medical school graduates at the same time, yet Carl Cori was employed as a researcher at the prestigious University of Vienna, Austria, and in the same capacity at Austria's University of Graz, whereas Gerty Cori was employed only as an assistant at a children's hospital (Karolinen) in 1920. In 1922, Carl Cori was hired as a biochemist at the New York State Institute for Study of Malignant Disease, yet Gerty Cori's position was only an assistant pathologist at the same institute. A further difference was when Carl Cori was offered the position of a professor and chairman of a department of pharmacology. Gerty Cori's employment was only a research fellow with a token salary. Gerty

Cori's publications were equal in number and significance to Carl's, but their employers took it for granted that Carl was superior to Gerty Cori. If she had not been awarded the Nobel Prize, her credit to science would be totally imbedded in Carl Cori's. While attitudes have changed, the important issue of sexual discrimination remains in scientific research.

16

RACHEL FULLER BROWN
(1898–1980)

Co-Discoverer of the Antifungal Antibiotic Nystatin .

If you have enough, why should you want more?—Rachel Fuller Brown
(1898–1980)

Rachel Fuller Brown co-discovered the first medically useful antifungal antibiotic nystatin with Elizabeth Hazen (1888–1975). These two devoted scientists refused to take any share of royalties from the patent rights for nystatin because they wanted all the money to be used for the advancement of science. Therefore, they established the Brown-Hazen Foundation funded by the royalties from the sale of this drug to support medical research, particularly research done by women scientists. The foundation also established many scholarships for the support of female students in the medical field. The life of Rachel Brown is an example of an American success story that demonstrates the best of human qualities.

Rachel Fuller Brown was born on November 23, 1898, in Springfield, Massachusetts. Her father was George Hamilton Brown, and her mother was Annie Fuller. Rachel had a younger brother. While Rachel was still a child, the whole family moved to Webster Groves, Missouri, where her father was a real estate and insurance agent. They lived there until she was 14 years old. During this period of her life, she and other children in her neighborhood came to know Professor Onderdonk who was a former high school principal from Albany, New York. He was interested in science and in young people. Rachel was interested in bugs and liked to collect every kind of insect in or near Webster Groves. Professor Onderdonk taught her how to use his microscope and preserve the specimens she collected. Rachel enjoyed seeing all kinds of things under Professor Onderdonk's microscope. This experience might have had some influence on her later development into a scientist.

Rachel's family wasn't a happy one. Her father left her mother, and

Rachel's mother moved the family back to Springfield, Massachusetts, in 1912 and raised Rachel and her brother alone. At this time she was ready to enter Central High School. In the high school years, she was a very good student and enjoyed all courses with no particular interest toward any subject. Unfortunately, the high school curriculum did not have chemistry or physics except for what was included in a semester course of general science. Rachel enjoyed performing some home experiments in chemistry, made possible by the gift of a Bunsen burner from an uncle.

Mrs. Brown was ambitious for her children and wanted them to go to college. She tried every way possible, including securing a loan and a scholarship. She also worked part-time and did whatever she could to help Rachel enter Mount Holyoke College in western Massachusetts, near Springfield, in 1916. Since Rachel didn't have much science background, she chose history as her college major.

Attending college wasn't easy despite the fact that Rachel had won a scholarship due to her excellent high school grades, and the cost was very high. Fortunately, a wealthy friend of Mrs. Brown's mother was impressed by Rachel's scholastic records and offered to assume complete responsibility for her college education. She helped so generously that Rachel had everything a Mount Holyoke student of her day could desire.

Not long after she started college, Rachel became deeply interested in chemistry. She said, "I liked it, though even today I can't be sure why, unless it was because of its ordered pattern and precision." She decided to add chemistry as a co-major. As a matter of fact, Mount Holyoke College had an excellent chemistry department headed by Dr. Emma Carr (1880–1972) at that time. Rachel Brown enjoyed her learning experience and received her A.B. degree in history and chemistry in 1920.

For advanced studies, armed with strong recommendation, Brown went to Dr. Carr's alma mater, the University of Chicago. She worked as a laboratory assistant and within a year, she received her master's degree in organic chemistry.

After getting the master's degree, Rachel began teaching in high school as did many young women at the time. She found a position at the Frances Shimer School in Chicago, which is a preparatory school and could be considered a junior college for girls. For three years, she taught physics and chemistry but discovered that she did not want to make a lifework out of this type of teaching. Having saved enough money, she returned to the University of Chicago in 1924 and worked on a Ph.D. degree in organic chemistry with a minor in bacteriology. She worked extremely hard and completed the course load in two years. The subject of her dissertation was the chemical properties of a pneumococcal-specific polysaccharide that could be used to identify one of the types of bacteria causing pneumonia. For reasons unknown to her, the acceptance of her dissertation was delayed, and the final oral examination was not scheduled. Therefore, her Ph.D. degree wasn't granted at that time.

Having run out of money and having assumed the responsibility of supporting her mother and grandmother, she accepted an offer as an assistant chemist in the Division of Laboratories and Research of the New York State Department of Health in Albany, New York. With her supervisor, Dr. Augustus B. Wadsworth (1872–1954), she developed a test to distinguish the unique polysaccharide coating on each type of pneumococcus. While attending a meeting in Chicago, she was contacted by her former professor at the University of Chicago who scheduled her final oral examination, which she readily passed. Her Ph.D. was finally granted in 1933.

Rachel Brown remained in Albany for 42 years. There she made distinguished accomplishments that benefited mankind. Rachel's primary job at Albany was to aid in diagnosing diseases from specimens sent by doctors and then in developing vaccines, antitoxins, and antisera for fighting the appropriate disease. This was the pre-antibiotics era, and developing antisera for fighting diseases was the mainstream of therapy. One of the top diseases of those days was pneumonia. Dr. Brown's first 15 years at Albany were spent working primarily on various facets of the chemistry of pneumococci. Dr. Brown extracted the specific carbohydrates from different pneumococci. These specific carbohydrates were used to identify the types of pneumococci. Eventually, more than forty types and many subtypes were studied. These carbohydrates could be used in standardizing the various pneumonia antisera prepared for distribution to physicians. There were many problems involved in the standardizing of these pneumonia antisera, and Dr. Brown contributed greatly to solving those problems. The specific type of pneumonia antiserum was used for the treatment of patients infected by that specific type of pneumococcus. When penicillin was discovered and proved effective against most types of pneumonia, pneumonia antisera lost their significance. Dr. Brown also worked on the chemistry of other microorganisms and published many papers in scientific journals. She was promoted to the rank of senior biochemist in 1936.

In addition to the assigned work, she had the freedom to work on other scientific problems of her interest. With the introduction of antibacterial antibiotics, Dr. Brown became interested in searching for antibiotics specifically effective for treating fungal infections, which often cause serious human maladies. Partly, this was inspired by the finding that antibiotics such as penicillin, streptomycin, chloromycetin, and chlorotetracycline were not only ineffective in fighting fungal infections in humans, but also might even encourage their development. For example, candidiasis, also known as moniliasis, caused by the yeast *Candida albicans*, is often encouraged by treatment with antibiotics. This fungus may cause lesions in the mouth, vagina, the skin, nails, bronchi, and lungs, and more rarely may cause a septicemia, an endocarditis, or a meningitis.

In the late 1940s, hunting for antibiotics to fight microbial infections was a main focus of research. Scientists at Brown's institution, led by Dr. Elizabeth Hazen (a mycologist), joined in the effort. Dr. Hazen had been hired by Dr. Wadsworth to work with Dr. Brown. Dr. Hazen had studied medical mycology at the College of Physicians and Surgeons of Columbia University in New York City. She set up a collection of disease-causing fungi, which were used to identify microorganisms in clinical specimens submitted by physicians around the state. In the search for antifungal antibiotics, Dr. Hazen investigated the actinomycetes (mold-like bacteria found mainly in soil). She collected many soil samples from everywhere in the world and isolated actinomycetes from these soils. She searched specifically for actinomycetes that were antagonistic to fungi known to cause human infections. A number of promising actinomycetes were found and she wanted to isolate the antifungal chemicals (antibiotics) from the cultured broth of these actinomycetes. Here started the fruitful cooperation with Dr. Rachel Brown, who was assigned, in 1948, by Dr. Gilbert Dalldorf (1900–1979), the new head of the division, to work with Dr. Hazen.

Dr. Hazen mainly worked at the New York City laboratory and Dr. Brown in Albany. Dr. Hazen cultured organisms found in soil samples and tested their activity *in vitro* against *Candida albicans* and *Cryptococcus neoformans*. When she found something interesting, she would mail active broth to Dr. Brown in Albany in mason jars. The high efficiency of sending the material by the U.S. Post Office in the 1940s also facilitated their discoveries.

Hazen had isolated and tested numerous actinomycetes and found good antifungal properties in two of them, No. 42705 and No. 48240 (later named *Streptomyces noursei*). But simply finding these properties was not enough. It was not uncommon for a promising culture to become worthless due to loss of activity upon cultivation or for an antibiotic to be degraded in the course of purification. It was also possible that a "new" antimicrobial agent had already been isolated previously and had been found to be too toxic for human use.

With Dr. Brown's enthusiastic effort and hard work, Dr. Hazen was able to isolate and purify one antibiotic from the pellicle of the actinomycete. This antibiotic was tentatively designated as fungicidin, a name that, unbeknownst to them at that time, had already been used for another substance. They also found another antibiotic from the culture broth and did not further purify it. They tested the effect of fungicidin against various kinds of fungi in experimental animals. They found that this antibiotic was effective against a large number of fungi and not effective against bacteria. Test on harmful fungi similar to some of those afflicting human beings had been promising. The results were announced at a New York State meeting of the National Academy of Sciences in early 1950. The announcement immediately attracted the attention of many pharmaceutical companies because they saw that Drs. Brown and Hazen had a patentable product that might have high commercial value. Since the help of the pharmaceutical industry was essential for further research and for testing, producing, and marketing a new product, Hazen and Brown turned to the Research Corporation for the handling of the patenting and licensing of the first effective, medically useful antifungal antibiotic. They decided to use the name nystatin instead of fungicidin because its first letters honored New York State in the laboratories in which the work had been done. E. R. Squibb and Sons helped to solve many problems related to commercial scale production. They helped develop a commercial version of the antibiotic that was first available in 1954. The US Patent (number 2,797,183) was issued on June 25, 1957.

Nystatin was proved nontoxic to human beings and could be administered alone or in combination with other antibiotics. Through its use, many illnesses from fungal infections were cured or prevented.

Some $135,000 royalties had been generated in the first year; more than $13 million would accrue before the patent expired. By an agreement between the Research Corporation and Brown and Hazen, all royalties were to be used to further research in the natural sciences. Half of them were distributed by grants made by the Research Corporation for the furtherance of investigations in scientific fields. The other half was distributed by the Brown-Hazen Fund for supporting fundamental studies in biochemistry, immunology, and microbiology, with special emphasis on affording advanced scientific training for the staff of the New York State Division of Laboratories and Research.

Dr. Brown continued to collaborate with Dr. Hazen to discover two other antibiotics, phalamycin and capacidin.

Brown received many awards and honors, including the Squibb Award in Chemotherapy in 1955, as well as honorary doctorate degrees from Hobart College, William Smith College, and Mount Holyoke College. She was given the Chemical Pioneer Award (with Dr. Hazen) from the American Institute of Chemists in 1975. Although she retired from the Division of Laboratories and Research in 1968 she remained involved in chemical research until her death on January 14, 1980, in Albany, New York.

Brown was a woman full of love toward her family as well as others. Her life outside the laboratory remained the same after her great discovery. She did, however, buy a comfortable, spacious home for her mother and grandmother. Brown was a member of St. Peter's Episcopal Church in Albany and was for many years a Sunday School teacher. She never married but had quite a church family. After the death of her grandmother, the empty bedroom was used as a guest room for a young Chinese physician who had been assigned to observe laboratory methods at the New York State Department of Health in Albany. The experience of sharing their home with a young Chinese woman was so rewarding that Dr. Brown and her mother considered themselves fortunate when a second Chinese woman, who was continuing her scientific work in Albany, took over the room just as its earlier occupant was leaving it. Since then, the Brown home was opened to all Chinese that it could accommodate. Beginning in 1946, her home was filled with Chinese students who returned to visit as often as a couple of times a year. For example, during Easter week of 1958, Brown noted that there were seven visiting Chinese who spent their vacation at the house. Dr. Brown said, "I just loved having them — I always do." She was especially fond of the children who had been born to members of the group here in America.

* * *

Nystatin is still widely used today to combat various fungal diseases such as ringworm and candidiasis. It has also been proved effective against fungal diseases of plants such as Dutch elm disease and against fungi that cause spoilage of bananas. It is also useful to protect paintings from fungal attack.

Dr. Brown was raised mainly by her mother who placed great emphasis on children's education. Mrs. Brown did everything possible to help Rachel to get a good education. Children who grow up in a family that respects education always have a better chance of becoming good citizens. One of Dr. Rachel Brown's accomplishments is a living witness of the importance of good education. Dr. Brown grew up in a poor family and carried heavy responsibilities, financial and otherwise, for others as well as for herself. However, she regarded her salary sufficient to provide her with a good life. She and Dr. Hazen refused to take any royalties from the discovery they made. She said, "If you have enough, why should you want more?" She spent every penny from the royalties on good causes. She was quite different from people who pursue money as the only purpose of life in today's world. Brown was always thankful to those who helped her. Since she received help from the benevolence of others, it was her lifelong objective to afford young people the kind of educational opportunity she had enjoyed.

Despite Dr. Brown's great scientific accomplishments, her final rank of associate biochemist was not attained until 1951, 15 years after her previous promotion. She was not even promoted to the level of full biochemist. She and Dr. Hazen were not recognized until very late in life, long after their great achievements. Although she shared with Dr. Hazen the Squibb Award in Chemotherapy in 1955, she and Dr. Hazen were not inducted into its legions in recognition of their contribution to medical science with their development of nystatin until 14 years (1994) after her death. Unfortunately, the scientific community seemed reluctant to reward woman scientists.

Further Reading

Bacon, W. S. 1976. Elizabeth Lee Hazen, 1888–1975. *Mycologia* (September/October): 961–969.

Oakes, Elizabeth H., ed. 2002. Rachel Fuller Brown (1898–1980). In *International Encyclopedia of Women Scientists*. New York: Facts on File. 44–45.

Yost, Edna, 1959. Rachel Fuller Brown (1898–). In *Women of Modern Science*. New York: Dodd, Mead. 64–79.

17

MARGARET PITTMAN
(1901–1995)

*Pioneer in Standardization of Biological Products
and Studies of Whooping Cough*

We may see but not perceive if the mind is not prepared. —Margaret Pittman
(1901–1995)

Margaret Pittman was a world renowned leader in medical microbiology. Her research involved the production, testing, and standardization of vaccines to prevent pertussis, cholera, typhoid, and other diseases. She studied the cause of whooping cough and contributed to the understanding of the pathogenesis of this disease. She was the first woman to be a director of a research laboratory at the National Institutes of Health. She also served as a consultant to the World Health Organization (WHO) for their cholera program.

The Pittmans came from England. They appeared in New England as early as 1653. In 1834, Samuel Pittman, the grandfather of Margaret, established a farm in Prairie Grove in a valley of the Ozark Mountains in northwest Arkansas. The stand of timber known as Prairie Grove was the site of a vicious battle in December 1862 during the Civil War. Margaret's father, James Pittman, was born in 1871 in a large cabin that later became the first post office in the valley. James was the first of seven children and received a good education at the University of Arkansas and St. Louis Medical College. He worked as a streetcar conductor to help defray family expenses during his school years. Margaret's mother, Virginia Alice McCormick, was also born in 1871 in Churchville in the Shenandoah Valley of Virginia. She was a cousin of Cyrus Hall McCormick (1809–1884), inventor of the harvester reaper. Her parents migrated via the Ohio, Mississippi, and Arkansas rivers to Evansville, Arkansas, in the Ozarks and finally settled in Prairie Grove, where they contracted typhoid fever and died. Virginia was a very talented person who, among other things, kept a lending library and taught the rudiments of piano. James and Virginia were married in 1899, and James began medical practice in Allen, which belonged to the Cherokee Nation of Oklahoma. Because they were afraid of malarial infections, they soon returned to Prairie Grove, where Margaret was born on January 20, 1901. Margaret had a sister, Helen, who became a public health nurse and later chair of the Department of Nursing at Sacred Heart Dominican College in Houston. She also had a brother, James, who became a general surgeon and chief of the surgical staff of Herman Hospital, Texas Medical Center, Houston. Their parents were good Christians and emphasized in their daily lives discipline, truth, love, education, and spiritual growth.

About 1909, the Pittman family moved to Cincinnati, Arkansas, 16 miles from Prairie Grove. Cincinnati was a country village, and James was the only doctor for miles around. He was a good doctor who responded to calls day or night, sunshine or rain. He was a true horse-and-buggy doctor who passionately served all people, even those who could not afford to pay. Margaret, even as a child, helped her father practice medicine. As Margaret recalled, her first medical experience was administration of anesthesia during the setting of a fractured bone. She also served as an assistant in vaccinating school children for smallpox in about ten rural schools. Smallpox vaccination was required by federal law at that time.

Margaret attended a very primitive school that had only two rooms. There she learned the fundamental subjects, but most importantly she developed the motivation to succeed. At home, Margaret and her siblings also received education from their parents who regarded a college education as essential. At night, by the glow of a kerosene lamp, they would read to the children current and classic novels in addition to the Bible.

Margaret attended high school for three years in Prairie Grove, where she stayed on her grandparents' farm. After high school, Margaret attended a newly organized college located in Siloam Springs, 12 miles north of Cincinnati. The college focused on music training and, because of long hours of piano practice, Margaret developed a spinal problem that plagued her for the rest of her life. Because of her illness and because she was not fond of playing piano, the music lessons were discontinued.

In 1919 Margaret's father died from peritonitis after an appendectomy, probably the victim of infected catgut used to sew his incision. Before his death, he requested that Margaret's mother take the three children to Hendrix College, a small accredited Methodist College in Conway, Arkansas. Her mother did so and supported her children's education by the creative use of her many talents, including canning vegetables and fruits in the summer.

At Hendrix, Margaret majored in mathematics and was such an outstanding student that she was awarded the college's Mathematics Medal. After one year, she was asked to teach a class in algebra. She also majored in biology and graduated *magna cum laude* in 1923. She was then offered a teaching position in the Academy of Galloway Female College in Searcy, Arkansas. She taught several subjects including science and Spanish. Starting as an instructor at $900 a year, she became principal of the academy in her second year with a salary of $1200 a year. After two years in that college, she decided to further her education by going to the University of Chicago.

Margaret was accepted as a graduate student, a candidate for the master's degree of science in the Department of Bacteriology and Hygiene. Bacteriology was a relatively new and exciting subject in biology. The department was created by Dr. Edwin Oakes Jordan (1866–1936), student of Dr. William Thompson Sedgwick (1855–1921). Margaret worked under the direction of Dr. I. S. Falk (1899–1984) on pneumococci and their pathogenicity. She completed the work and published a paper entitled "Studies on Respiratory Diseases XXXIV: Some Relations between Extracts, Filtrates and Virulence of Pneumococci" in the *Journal of Bacteriology* in 1930.

After receiving her master's degree, she was offered a fellowship to continue her studies toward a Ph.D. degree. The fellowship was from the Influenza Commission of the Metropolitan Life Insurance Company and paid $75.00 per month. She took many valuable courses such as biochemistry, human anatomy and dissection, histology, and pathology at the University of Chicago Medical School. She also did research under the direction of Professor Mercy A. Southwith in the Department of Pathology. In 1929 she completed her Ph.D. dissertation entitled *Pathology of Experimental Pneumococcus Lobar Pneumonia.*

In the fall of 1928 (before her Ph.D. degree was granted), Margaret was offered a postdoctoral position by Dr. Rufus Cole (1872–1966), director of the Hospital of the Rockefeller Institute for Medical Research (RIH). (The Rockefeller Institute is the forerunner of Rockefeller University.) At RIH, she had the opportunity to be associated with the Acute Respiratory Group led by Dr. O. T. Avery (1877–1955). She worked on *Haemophilus influenzae* and other microorganisms relevant to influenza and other diseases. She discovered that the capsules of *H. influenzae* and the "S" and "R" colonies of *H. influenzae* were similar to those of the pneumococci. In less than four years at RIH, she identified the six serotypes (a, b, c, d, e and nontypable) among 521 hemophilic strains of *H. influenzae* isolated largely from the sputa of pneumonia patients admitted to RIH. Only a few isolated strains were encapsulated, and type b was dominant and the most pathogenic. She discovered that strains associated with influenza were not encapsulated. She demonstrated that strains of *H. influenzae* from meningitis patients were usually of type b. She also demonstrated that type b antiserum had therapeutic value. This research was published in 1931 and received worldwide attention. Dr. Pittman became an internationally known scientist at only 30 years of age. Later it was discovered that type b carbohydrates conjugated with a protein antigen that would contribute to the prevention of the type b infection.

Dr. Pittman's work on the characteristics of more than 500 hemophilic cultures relevant to the incidence of encapsulated strains led her to become an expert on the taxonomy of the genus of Haemophilus. She was invited to prepare the section "Genus Haemophilus Winslow et al. 1917" for *Bergey's Manual of Determinative Bacteriology*, edition 5 (1939), 6 (1948), and 7 (1957). In the seventh edition, *H. aegyptius* was listed as a separate species. The organism *Haemophilus pertussis*, which Dr. Pittman studied extensively, was put into the genus *Bordetella* in 1988.

Dr. Pittman had also isolated the Koch-Weeks bacillus (now called *Haemophilus aegyptius*) and the influenza bacillus (*Haemophilus influenzae*) from children with conjunctivitis. The colony of *H. aegyptius* in semi-solid media was small and fluffy with a comet-like tail. The colony of non-typable *H. influenzae* was small and granular, while the colony of encapsulated bacteria was large and fluffy. *Haemophilus aegyptius* is limited to the conjunctiva and occurs only during hot weather, whereas, *H. influenzae* infection occurs anywhere in the eye.

Dr. Pittman's service at the RIH ended in 1934 when the economic depression gripped the United States. She took a position with a salary cut at the New York State Department of Health Laboratories, where she prepared biological products and engaged in laboratory diagnoses for a year and a half.

In 1902 the United States Congress passed the Congressional Biologics Control Act. The purpose of the act was to ensure the continued safety, purity, and potency of all vaccines, toxins, antitoxins, therapeutics and sera, or analogous products applicable to the prevention, treatment, and cure of disease or injuries. The National Institutes of Health (NIH) was designated to regulate the Control Act. The responsibility was transferred to the Food and Drug Administration in 1972.

In 1936 Dr. Pittman was employed by NIH to work with Dr. Sara E. Branham (1888–1962), one of her former professors at the University of

Chicago. Their first assignment was to develop a potency test for meningo-coccus antisera. Dr. Pittman developed a precipitin test for the specific meningococcus antibodies. The test was later used for the isolation of *H. influenzae* and *Salmonella typhi*. She then studied the *Neisseria meningitidis* and *H. influenzae* in 1937. Dr. Pittman had done a lot of research on the potency assay and the precipitin test. She developed the badly needed stan-dards for the efficacy for type b *H. influenzae* antisera and *Bordella pertussis* antisera.

During this period of time, she conducted an extensive study on the pyrogenicity of plasma and its contaminants. The pyrogenicity of plasma was due to the presence of microorganisms in distilled water. She found that all microorganisms were capable of inducing fever but that Gram-negative bacteria were most pyrogenic. One ml of water containing 6000 col-ony forming units (CFU) was sufficient to induce pyrogenicity. Following their work, a rabbit pyrogenicity test was applied to all intravenous fluid products.

She also examined the sterility of biological products. She was involved in the development of the fluid thioglycolate medium (FTM), which was later used by the World Health Organization (WHO) for detection of both aerobic and anaerobic contaminant of biological substances. She found that the methylene blue oxidation reduction indicator in the medium inhib-ited growth of some organisms, which were found as contaminants in blood and blood products. The formula for the medium was revised by substitu-tion of resazurin as the indicator and by addition of cysteine to better sup-port the growth of anaerobes. In addition, she developed the inclusion of a medium for the detection of fungal contaminants in biological products. Dr. Pittman also studied the contaminants of blood and provided a better under-standing of the problems of bacterial contamination in the handling of blood and blood products. She was extensively involved with the development of potency assays of pertussis, typhoid, and cholera vaccines and participated in the study of the correlation of potency with human efficacy of these prod-ucts.

The first trial of pertussis antiserum therapy was done by Jules Bordet (1870–1961) and Octave Gengou in 1909. Since then pertussis vaccines have been widely used. Early in the vaccine assay, Dr. John F. Norton of Upjohn Company discovered that mice could be infected intracerebrally with *Borde-tella pertussis* and that they could be protected by pertussis vaccine. Dr. Pittman persistently studied the pertussis vaccine. She and Dr. Pearl Kendrick of Michigan State Bureau of Laboratories tried the intracerebral route of chal-lenges in the potency testing of pertussis vaccine. As a result of many tests, the standards for the pertussis vaccine were established in 1949. Dr. Pittman discovered that alum adjuvant influenced the toxicity of the vaccine. With Dr. Maria G. Stronk, she found that the mouse strain used for testing was also critical. She reported the unreliability of standardizing vaccines based solely on the number of organisms or on turbidity of the vaccines and applied statistical methods to estimate the efficacy dosage (ED_{50}) of the vaccines. She also studied extensively the antigenicity and toxicity of the vaccines, particularly the role of pertussis toxin in whooping cough. She and Dr. Stronk illustrated the molecular structure of pertussis toxin and its activity affected by catalytic action of ADP–ribosyltransferase. Her contribution to the understanding and standardization of pertussis vaccine has been tremendous.

In 1958 Dr. Pittman participated in the development of the first international requirements for biological substances — yellow fever vaccine and cholera vaccine. In 1959 the requirements for cholera vaccine were published. Other meetings with the World Health Organization (WHO) and cooperative tests followed. Dr. Pittman was involved with the Cholera Research Laboratory in Decca, East Pakistan (now Bangladesh). She later served for about five years as NIH project director of the Cholera Research Laboratory. Her interest was the relationship of the laboratory potency assay to efficacy of the cholera vaccine. Eventually it was shown that the mouse potency assay of the cholera vaccine was directly related to the effectiveness of the vaccine in field trials.

Likewise, Dr. Pittman participated in the laboratory assessment of the potency of typhoid vaccines that were tested in WHO field trials. Her work contributed to promulgation of the U.S. Standards for typhoid fever vaccines. She and her colleagues made a great contribution to the understanding of the importance of Vi antigen, which is present in the typhoid organism, *Salmonella typhi*, in human immunity. She was also involved with Dr. F. D. Schofield and Dr. R. MacLennon in an extensive study on "Immunization against Neonatal Tetanus in New Guinea," which led to the successful prevention of neonatal tetanus with tetanus toxoid vaccine. Additionally, Dr. Pittman participated in the testing of other bacterial products such as guinea pig skin potency assay that was included in the first requirements for tuberculins. She also worked on requirements for anthrax vaccine and vaccines to prevent *Clostridium* gangrene that have limited use.

Dr. Pittman was promoted to Chief, Laboratory of Bacterial Products, a Division of Biologics Standards in 1957. She was the first woman to be named chief of an NIH laboratory. During 1967–1970, she was a guest lecturer at Howard University College of Medicine in Washington, D.C.

Dr. Pittman remained at NIH until 1971 when she officially retired. After that she was a guest worker without official responsibility or pay. She continued to do research, completing pending manuscripts, presenting invited lectures, participating in workshops, and writing articles for journals and books.

Dr. Pittman was a consultant or guest scientist in nine countries. With WHO, she completed the revision of requirements for the sterility test of biological substances and was a consultant on cholera vaccination in Cairo, Egypt, and Madrid, Spain. She served as a consultant to the Board of Directors of Connaught Laboratories, Ltd., Toronto, Canada, and from December 1974 to March 1975, she was a consultant to the State Institute for Serum and Vaccine in Raz, Teheran, Iran.

She continued her investigation on the role of pertussis toxin in the pathogenicity of whooping cough. In collaboration with Professor A. C. Wardlaw of the University of Glasgow, Scotland, where she was a visiting scientist and consultant, and Dr. Brian L. Furman of the University of Strathclyde, Glasgow, she demonstrated that pertussis toxin (a true exotoxin, the histamine sensitizing factor) is the cause of the harmful effects. The toxin can also prolong immunity of whooping cough and the pathophysiological reactions of the mouse infected with *B. pertussis* by the intra-nasal route. These were great contributions to the understanding of the disease of whooping cough. She published more than twenty additional papers after her retirement.

Dr. Pittman was active in serving many professional societies. She was a member of the American Society for Microbiology (ASM), serving as Councilor 1955–1956 and 1958–1960, and president of the Washington, D.C. branch, 1949–1950. She was on the Board of Governors of the American Academy of Microbiology from 1963 to 1969. She was a diplomat of the American Board of Microbiology and in 1976 was made an honorary member of ASM. She served on numerous committees of the Washington Academy of Sciences and was its first woman president in 1955.

In the international scene, she was a U.S. delegate to the Fifth International Microbiology Congress in Rio de Janeiro in 1950. She participated in the conference on whooping cough at the International Children's Center in Paris in 1957 and was a member of two WHO study groups held in Geneva, Switzerland, for the formulation of International Recommended Requirements for Biological Substances (cholera vaccine and yellow fever vaccine in 1958, and sterility in 1959). In 1962 she was a WHO consultant at the Biological Standardization Conference on Pertussis Vaccine in Geneva. In the same year, she also participated in the conference on whooping cough in

Prague, Czechoslovakia. She was a member of the NIH Cholera Advisory Committee and a member of the Panel of Expert Consultants to the Technical Committee for Pakistan-Southeast Asia Treaty Organization (SEATO) Cholera Research Laboratory, Dacca. She also organized the Pertussis Vaccine Symposium sponsored by NIH Division of Biological Standards (DBS) in 1963. Additionally, she also served on the Armed Forces Epidemiological Board, Commission on Immunization. She actively participated in the United States Pharmacopoeia Advisory Panel on Sterility Tests and Standardization Procedure (1967–1970) and on Biological Indicators (1970–1973).

Numerous honors and awards have been bestowed upon Dr. Pittman. She was awarded an honorary LL.D. in 1954 by Hendrix College. She has been listed *in American Men and Women of Science* since 1936 and was first listed in *Who's Who* in 1960. In 1963 she received a Superior Service Award from the Department of Health, Education, and Welfare (DHEW), and Distinguished Service Award from DHEW in 1967. In 1970 she received the Federal Women's Award. In 1973 the University of Chicago Alumni Association awarded her the Professional Achievement Award. She was made honorary member of Sigma Delta Epsilon in 1974.

Dr. Pittman was a travel enthusiast. She had ample opportunity to see the world in her official capacity, but she often extended those trips for personal interest and pleasure. For example, in the interest of studying cholera, she visited Bangkok, Taiwan, Calcutta, Bombay, and the Philippines. After attending the International Microbiological Congress in Rio de Janeiro in 1950, she visited most of the countries in South America. Following professional visits to Iran, she visited Teheran, Isfahan, and Shiraz as side trips. She even visited the Abadan area and sites of the Elamite civilization including Sushan.

Dr. Pittman was a member of the Mount Vernon United Methodist Church of Washington, D.C., and was active in a number of church activities. She once served as chairperson of the church finance committee that formulated successful plans for paying off a $200,000 debt. She was also a member of the Board of Trustees and chaired the Pastor Parish Relations Committee.

*   *   *

From her family background, with home training and inspirational education, Dr. Pittman was a woman with a great heart. She expressed a high interest in different civilizations and cultures. She had a great global viewpoint in her work, as well as a strong compassion.

Dr. Pittman worked in an era where women were still a minority in the scientific community. She admitted to no discrimination in her career as a woman. She never asked for a promotion. Her promotions were totally deserved due to her performance. She always praised her staff for their high *esprit de corps* and their outstanding research contributions. She expressed her impatience with women who expected too much too soon with too little preparation.

Dr. Margaret Pittman was never married but lived a full rewarding life. She passed away in 1995. Her work continues to save many lives, and her compassion also inspires many young minds.

18

VIRGINIA APGAR
(1909–1974)

Pioneer Anesthetist and Developer of
the Apgar Score for Newborn Health

Women were liberated from the time they were born.—Virginia Apgar
(1909–1974)

Virginia Apgar developed a test called Apgar Score System, which was designed to evaluate the health of newborns. This score system helped save the lives of many infants and became a standard procedure in hospitals worldwide. Apgar also made numerous contributions in obstetric anesthesia, which benefited the raising of healthy children.

Virginia Apgar was born on June 7, 1909, in Westfield, New Jersey. Her father was Charles Emory Apgar (1865–1950), and her mother was Helen Clarke. Charles was a salesman for the New York Life Insurance Company and also an executive for Spencer Trask & Company. Charles had many hobbies including astronomy and wireless telegraphy. He was a successful amateur scientist, making his home basement a laboratory where he did experiments with electricity and radio waves. He also built a telescope for his astronomical work. His research endeavors resulted in several scientific papers, which were published in the *Royal Canadian Astronomical Society*. In 1915 Charles operated a private radio station, W2MN. During World War I, Charles helped the War Department crack the message about the movements of neutral ships in a secret code sent from the German station at Sayville, Long Island, to German submarines.

Charles' scientific hobbies might have influenced Virginia to become interested in science. After graduation from high school, Virginia had already determined to be a medical doctor. No specific events seem to have triggered her decision. She did not meet a woman doctor in her childhood, nor did she have any serious illness. However, an older brother, Charles Emory Apgar,

Jr. (1900–1904), had died of tuberculosis at age three, and another brother, Lawrence C. Apgar (1907–1988), had childhood eczema, which caused him to frequently visit the family doctor. The family medical history might have had some impact on her decision to become a doctor.

In the 1920s Virginia entered Mount Holyoke College, South Hadley, Massachusetts. She was a very active student. She worked very hard as a waitress, and assistant in the school library, and a technician for the zoological laboratory, and did various other jobs in order to pay her tuition. She was also involved in many extracurricular activities such as writing for the college newspaper, playing in the orchestra, participating in the theater, and playing tennis. After graduation in 1929, she entered the College of Physicians and Surgeons at Columbia University, New York. During her school years, although she had a small scholarship, she had to borrow money from family friends in order to support herself. The stockmarket crashed in October of 1929 and the Great Depression began; it was a difficult period for everybody including the Apgar family. Virginia struggled through these difficulties and graduated fourth in her class in addition to being elected a member of Alpha Omega Alpha in 1933. However, at this time, she was $4,000 in debt.

Apgar was determined to become a surgeon and obtained a prized surgical internship at Columbia when she performed brilliantly and seemed headed toward a bright future as a surgeon. However, Dr. Alan Whipple (1881–1963), chairman of surgery, discouraged her from continuing to pursue a career in surgery. Instead, he encouraged her to investigate anesthesiology, a new field in medicine. There were sufficient reasons for Dr. Whipple to do so because he had trained four other women surgeons, and they had not been financially successful. There was a surplus of surgeons in New York City at the time, but there was a need for better anesthesiologists. Dr. Whipple realized that surgery could not advance unless anesthesia did, and most importantly, he recognized the intelligence, energy, and ability of Apgar, who could make significant contributions in this area.

It was also possible that Whipple thought that anesthesiology was particularly suitable for a woman. Most anesthesia at the time was given by nurse anesthetists, a practice dating to the 1880s. The nurse anesthetists were reliable, patient, and technically skilled but lacked the more complete training of women physicians who would have the same "feminine" traits in addition to medical training. Whipple advised Apgar to look to anesthesiology instead of surgery as a career. In 1934 Apgar accepted this advice and began her search for proper training. She wrote to Dr. Francis H. McMechan (1879–1939), secretary-general of the Associated Anesthetists of the United States and Canada, requesting a list of possible training positions.

Apgar's road to becoming a successful anesthetist was somewhat bumpy. After finishing her surgical internship in November 1935, Apgar stayed for a while at Columbia to work with the head nurse anesthetist. Wanting to gain more experience of anesthesia, she went to Madison, Wisconsin, on January 1, 1937, to work with Dr. Ralph Waters (1883–1979) in the department of anesthesiology at the University of Wisconsin School of Medicine, the first and most important anesthesiology department in the country. But she suffered from a common problem of women physicians working in hospitals at the time: lack of housing facilities. She had to move three times in six months. In July she returned to New York City to work with Dr. Ernest Rovenstine at Bellevue Hospital. Again, she faced housing problems. She had to stay in the clinic building's maids' quarters, and she felt excluded from male medical activities. She wrote in her diary, "Fairly good meeting but stag dinner — MAD!"

In 1938 after another six months at Bellevue, she returned to Columbia as Director of the Division of Anesthesia and Attending Anesthetist Assigned at Presbyterian Hospital. She successfully built a solid anesthesiology department with excellent research productivity. She encountered numerous problems; for example, the recruitment of physicians was not easy because anesthesia was still considered a nurse's job and the clinical load was overwhelming. Many male physicians entered the armed services because of World War II (1941–1945). Apgar was the only staff member until August 1940, when Dr. Ellen Foot joined her as a resident. The surgeons were reluctant to accept physician anesthesiologists as their equals in the operating room because surgeons previously had to administer anesthesia. They were accustomed to giving the anesthetists orders and were slow at recognizing that the practice of anesthesia had changed. Also it was difficult for the anesthesiologists to receive adequate compensation because physicians giving anesthesia were not allowed to charge professional fees. Apgar fought seriously to change many unreasonable rules, and she solved many problems including setting proper fees for services rendered by her profession. A new division of anesthesiology was formed at Columbia in 1949, but Apgar, against expectation, was not named chair because she was considered lacking sophisticated research training. Dr. Emmanuel Papper (1915–2002), a Bellevue anesthesiologist with a research background, was made head of the division. The new division became a department six months later. Both Apgar and Papper were appointed professors.

From then on, Apgar was freed from the frustration of administration and devoted herself wholeheartedly to the anesthesia research. As a result, she made a milestone contribution to children's preventive medicine. Before

Apgar's time, there was no standard evaluation of the health of newborn infants, who were generally taken directly from the delivery room to the hospital nursery. Because of the cursory treatment given to the newborns, health problems generally were not noticed until they became critical or fatal. Apgar developed a simple test, which came to be known as the Apgar Score System. In this system, a scale ranging from zero to two was used to evaluate the newborn's skin color, muscle tone, breathing, heart rate, and reflexes. The resultant total score indicated the physical conditions of infants. A low score was indicative of problems requiring immediate attention, while a high score indicated a healthy baby. This Apgar Score System was presented at the annual meeting of the American Society of Anesthesiologists in 1952 and was published in 1953. As with any new invention, there was some resistance initially, but eventually this system was accepted and used throughout the world.

The significance of the score system was that the newborn infant could be observed in a standard multifaceted way within a minute of delivery. Initially, the score system was to be done within one minute after birth so that it could be a guide to the need for resuscitation. Apgar emphasized that physicians should not wait the entire one minute to complete the score before resuscitating an obviously depressed baby. Later, nurses measured the score at longer intervals after birth to evaluate how the baby was responding to any necessary resuscitation. Now, the one-minute and five-minute Apgar score tests are standard practice.

Apgar went on to investigate the relationship between the newborn baby's acid-base status and the anesthetics administered to the mother. The research was in collaboration with Dr. L. Stanley James (1925–1994), a pediatrician from New Zealand, and Dr. Duncan A. Holaday (1902–1989), who had been trained in anesthesiology and did research at Johns Hopkins University. Holaday developed a nitrogen washout technique for measuring the general anesthetic cyclopropane, used the Nadelson microgasometer to measure arterial blood gases in the presence of anesthetics, and developed a better pH measurement method. It is also worthy to point out that the Astrup pH electrode available in 1960 made pH measurement easier and helped tremendously in this study.

With the help from these researchers and the availability of new technology, Apgar discovered that hypoxic, acidotic babies were found to have low Apgar scores. The acidosis and hypoxia were not normal conditions at birth as was previously thought and should be treated. She was also the first person to catheterize the umbilical artery of the newborn when she and L. Stanley James investigated changes in venous pressure after birth by passing catheters into the right atrium through the umbilical vein.

They also investigated the effects of anesthetics used on the baby. When they found that cyclopropane was more depressant than other agents, the use of cyclopropane in obstetrics was discouraged and thus decreased markedly. With the collaborative efforts of 12 institutions that involved 17,221 babies, Apgar and James established that the Apgar score, especially the five-minute score, was a reliable predictor of neonatal survival and of future neurological development.

After many years of research, Apgar felt the need to return to school. She went to Johns Hopkins University to learn more about statistics in order to effectively evaluate her studies. She eventually received a master's degree in public health in 1959. In the same year, she accepted the position of senior executive with the National Foundation (previously the March of Dimes) in their new division of congenital defects. She was enormously successful in raising funds to support research on infants' defects and to increase public support and awareness. She eventually became the director of the organization's research department. She held this position until her death of liver disease in 1974 at the age of 65.

Several honors and awards were bestowed upon Apgar. She received the Elizabeth Blackwell Citation from the New York Infirmary in 1960, the Distinguished Service Award of the American Society of Anesthesiologists in 1961, and the Gold Medal for Distinguished Achievement in Medicine awarded by Columbia University's College of Physicians and Surgeons in 1973. She was also named Woman of the Year in Science by *Ladies' Home Journal* in 1973. In 1994 she was honored with a U.S. stamp in her name. Apgar was the only anesthesiologist and the third woman physician to be honored with a U.S. stamp. On October 14, 1995, she was inducted into the National Women's Hall of Fame in Seneca Falls, New York.

A musician since childhood, Apgar often carried her cello or viola on her frequent travels and joined chamber music groups for a night of playing in cities she visited.

Apgar was also a maker of stringed musical instruments. Her interest in constructing stringed instruments started in 1956 when she visited Mrs. Carleen Hutchings, a high school science teacher and musician. Mrs. Hutchings had built her own violin and when she was in the hospital for surgery, she invited Dr. Apgar during the preoperative visit to play her homemade violin. Apgar was enchanted by the excellent quality of sound of the instrument and became interested in learning instrument construction from her. Eventually, she built four stringed instruments of her own: a violin, a mezzo violin, a cello, and a viola.

In order to make good musical instruments, she always looked for suitable fine wood to use. In 1957 Mrs. Hutchings found an excellent piece of curly maple used as a shelf in a pay telephone booth in the lobby of the Harkness Pavilion of Columbia-Presbyterian Medical Center. Of course, since it was not possible to get the shelf through regular channels of the hospital bureaucracy, Apgar and Mrs. Hutchings plotted a direct but an extraordinary way to get the shelf of curly maple. This was later referred to as the "phone booth caper" and was eventually reported in the *New York Times* on February 2, 1975. Dr. Apgar stained a piece of wood to match the one in the phone booth. Fortunately, it was possible to obtain the very stain from the hardware store near the hospital that supplied the original stain to the hospital 27 years earlier. When everything was ready, Mrs. Hutchings began her work in the phone booth late at night with Apgar dressed in her hospital uniform, standing guard in the hall. When the night watchman came by on his rounds, Dr. Apgar would tap on the door of the booth, and Mrs. Hutchings would put a dime in the phone to pretend to make a call. Things were going fine, but the planning had not been perfected. Mrs. Hutchings found that her substitute shelf was a quarter of an inch too long. Undisturbed, she went to the women's restroom with her saw while Dr. Apgar stood guard. A passing nurse was somewhat surprised to hear a sawing noise coming from the women's restroom. Dr. Apgar stated loudly, "It's the only time the repairman can work in there." The nurse was satisfied with that explanation and the plan was a success. The removed shelf went on to enjoy a new life as the back of Apgar's viola.

The four instruments handcrafted by Dr. Apgar were played by a string quartet, the "Apgar String Quartet," in October 1994, when the stamp honoring Dr. Apgar was released at the American Academy of Pediatrics' annual meeting in Dallas, Texas. The quartet was made up of four pediatricians: Nick Cunningham, M.D. (cello), Mary Howell, M.D. (mezzo violin), Yeou-Cheng Ma, M.D. (first violin; she is cellist Yo-Yo Ma's sister), and Robert Levine, M.D. (viola). They played Dr. Apgar's favorite chamber music at two events: a luncheon during which the 20th Annual Virginia Apgar Award in Perinatal Medicine was awarded, and the stamp's unveiling ceremony.

These four instruments have been donated to Columbia University and are now available for rental. Music was a vital part of Dr. Apgar's life, and Dr. Apgar's life was like wonderful music, which enlightened many lives.

*   *   *

Apgar devoted her life to the welfare of infants. She could have been a good surgeon had she insisted on pursuing that career, but she entered anesthesiology instead because of the need of anesthesiologists in her time. She was an enthusiastic, hard working, and prepared physician. When opportunity arose, she grasped it and was rewarded with success.

Was she not aware of the gender discrimination against her in her career? She certainly was. She recognized clearly the lack of equal opportunity for her as a woman physician, but she battled with professional competency and overcame all the restrictions. She could have been an excellent departmental chair, but she was not offered the opportunity mainly because she was a female. Instead of fighting for equal opportunity, she entered research in obstetric anesthesia because there was a great need. She took the advantage of freeing herself from administration and industriously engaged in research, where she made great contributions. She often said that "women were liberated from the time they were born." She never participated in female medical organizations, because she felt she did not need them. But she fully recognized that women were not given the same opportunities. In her diary, she expressed outrage at such things as salary differentials between her and her male colleagues and the "stag" dinners that followed professional meetings. She overcame the restrictions limiting her and took advantages of the available opportunities to make an outstanding career. She was indeed a role model for all women and beautiful music to all mankind.

Further Reading

Anesthesia service in hospital. 1940. *Journal of the American Medical Association* 114: 1260–1261.

Apgar, Virginia. Interview. Box 1, Folder 1, Apgar Papers, Mt. Holyoke College Library Archives.

_____. Record of expenses, 1929–1937. Box 10, Apgar Papers, Mt. Holyoke College Library Archives.

Calmes, S. H. 1984. Virginia Apgar: a woman physician's career in a developing specialty. *Journal of the American Medical Women's Association* 39(6): 184–188.

Duncum, B. 1947. *The Development of Inhalation Anesthesia.* New York: Oxford University Press.

Rappleye, Willard C. Letter to Virginia Apgar, 7 June 1933. Box 5, Folder 21, Apgar Papers, Mount Holyoke College Library Archives.

Sullivan, W. 1975. Confessions of a musical shelf-robber. *New York Times*, Feb. 2.

19

GLADYS LOUNSBURY HOBBY
(1910–1993)

Leader in the Study of Antibiotics and Anti-Tuberculosis Drugs

Terramycin is a trade name of the antibiotic oxytetracycline, which has been widely used in fighting rickettsial, chlamydial, mycoplasmal, and some fungal infections. This miracle drug was discovered by Gladys Lounsbury Hobby, who was a leader in the studies of antibiotics. She was involved in the beginning of critical research on penicillin, streptomycin, viomycin, and the broad spectrum of antibiotics. She also contributed to the chemotherapy of tuberculosis. She is certainly a woman of distinction whose story is worthwhile for us to learn.

Gladys Lounsbury Hobby was born on November 19, 1910, in Washington Heights in New York City. Her father was Theodore Y. Hobby, and her mother was Flora Lounsbury Hobby. Flora Lounsbury Hobby was a school teacher and taught in the New York City public school system. Theodore Hobby was initially in the retail dry goods business and later became a close associate of Mr. Benjamin Altman, who collected porcelain, paintings, and other works of art that ultimately comprised the Altman Collection at the Metropolitan Museum of Art in New York City. Mr. Hobby traveled frequently with Mr. Altman in Europe and became "keeper" of the Altman Collection at the Museum. He also became associate curator of Far Eastern Art and helped Mr. John D. Rockefeller II in collecting Japanese and Chinese porcelains. These porcelain objects are now part of the Rockefeller Collection at the Metropolitan Museum of Art in New York. Although Gladys was interested in science and had a career in scientific research, she acquired an appreciation of art from her parents at a young age.

Gladys was a smart student. She attended the upper grades and high school in White Plains in New York and later attended Vassar College, where she first learned bacteriology from Dr. Anne Benton Riebeth. While still in college she worked under Dr. Anna Williams (1863–1954) and Dr. Annis Thomas at the New York City Department of Health Laboratories. This training initiated her interest in bacteriology. Following graduation in 1931, she continued her study of bacteriology at the College of Physicians and Surgeons at Columbia University in New York. She worked on *Corynebacterium diphtheriae*, the cause of diphtheria, and obtained her M.S. degree in 1932 and a Ph.D. degree in 1935. In her dissertation, Gladys applied the phenomenon of microbial variation as described by Joseph A. Arkwright (1864–1944), Frederick Griffith (1879–1941), and Martin Henry Dawson (1896–1945) to study the diphtheria bacillus. She was also interested in Dr. Dawson's work on rheumatic fever.

In 1934 Gladys moved from the Bacteriology Department at the College of Physicians and Surgeons to the Department of Medicine to work with Dr. Dawson. Gladys worked closely with Dr. Dawson and collaborated with Rebecca Lancefield (1895–1981) on the morphological, serological, and disease-producing properties of hemolytic streptococci. Dr. Dawson's interest in rheumatic disease brought them in contact with many patients with subacute bacterial endocarditis, which is often fatal. Dr. Hobby developed a strong desire to find a cure for this disease. Therefore, she was interested in experimental chemotherapy. She began to use gold salts, the sulfonamides, and finally penicillin. The miracle drug penicillin was discovered by Alexander Fleming (1881–1955) at St. Mary's Hospital in London, England, in 1928, but its clinical potential was not appreciated at the time. Under the leadership of Dr. Dawson and the collaboration of Dr. Karl Meyer (b.1899), a chemist at the College of Physicians and Surgeons, Gladys prepared the first penicillin made in the United States. In 1940 Dr. Dawson initiated the first clinical trials of the chemotherapeutic action of penicillin and tested it successfully on a patient with subacute bacterial endocarditis. For Dr. Gladys Hobby, this was the beginning of many years of research on antimicrobial drugs.

Drs. Hobby, Dawson, and Meyer, who worked as a team, demonstrated the chemotherapeutic potential of penicillin and investigated the relationship between the infectious dose and the amount of penicillin required to protect experimentally infected animals. Additionally, they showed that penicillin was effective only against actively growing microbial cells. Following these studies in animals, Drs. Dawson and Hobby made a detailed study of the clinical effectiveness of penicillin, and between 1940 and 1944 they reported the therapeutic effect of the drug in 100 patients. Following Dr. Dawson's death in 1945, Dr. Hobby moved to Chas Pfizer & Co., Inc., to continue the research. Their work made penicillin a useful antibiotic to treat many diseases.

Dr. Hobby continued her research on antimicrobial agents for 15 years at Pfizer (1944–1959). Within five years at Pfizer, she was co-discoverer of oxytetracycline (brand name Terramycin). She organized the experimental evaluation and the clinical trials of the drug. Dr. Hobby prepared the new drug application for its approval by the United States Food and Drug Administration. She also traveled extensively throughout the United States and many foreign countries to promote the use of the drug.

The tetracycline antibiotics are effective against many different types of bacteria. They control Gram-positive and Gram-negative bacteria, chlamydia, rickettsiae, and mycoplasmas. The mode of action of tetracycline antibiotics was to interfere with bacterial protein synthesis by blocking the ribosomes' acceptance of aminoacyl-tRNA. Because tetracycline antibiotics were easy to administer orally and had an extremely broad spectrum, they were widely used clinically. They were also added to animal feed to enhance the growth of livestock. However, they were later found to have side effects such as gastrointestinal pain and irritation by dramatically changing the normal microbiota of the intestine. They also caused increased sensitivity to sunlight and caused teeth to develop brown stains. Now, tetracycline drugs are used only to treat acne and infections caused by chlamydia, rickettsiae, and mycoplasmas.

During the early years at Pfizer, Dr. Hobby also had an academic appointment at Columbia University where she taught bacteriology. However, because she had to travel extensively for the promotion of Terramycin, she resigned her academic position. Shortly after leaving Pfizer, she was appointed clinical instructor (1959–1973) and later clinical assistant professor (1974–1977) of public health at Cornell Medical College in New York.

Dr. Hobby was a leader in the study of antimicrobial agents. In 1951 she published an historical review of microbiology in relation to antibiotics, in which she pointed out the serendipity in Fleming's observations and how fortuitous a discovery it was that penicillin was the first antibiotic studied. She discussed the drug's availability, its spectrum of action, and its bactericidal effect on sensitive organisms as well as its low toxicity — all positive factors leading to the clinical use of penicillin.

In 1959 Dr. Hobby accepted the appointment as Chief of the Veterans Administration Special Research Laboratory for the study of Chronic Infectious Diseases located in East Orange, New Jersey. She continued her research for another 18 years (1959–1977). She devoted her research efforts primarily to the control of tuberculosis, which is and has been throughout history one of the most widely distributed and deadly diseases affecting humans. She studied extensively each of the many antituberculous drugs that were introduced. She evaluated the extent and significance of the emergence of the resistance of tubercle bacilli (*Mycobacterium tuberculosis*) to antimicrobial agents. She demonstrated clearly that the antibacterial drug streptomycin, with or without *p*-aminosalicylic acid, was not sufficient to eradicate viable tubercle bacilli from tuberculous lesions in human patients.

Dr. Hobby's work has contributed greatly to the control of the incidence of tuberculosis in the United States and the world. However, tuberculosis remains the leading killer among all infectious diseases, with an estimated 10 million new cases and 3 million deaths annually. Tuberculosis accounts for about a quarter of avoidable adult deaths. The major concern today is the appearance of new strains of *M. tuberculosis* that are resistant to most currently available drugs. The current spread of AIDS also contributes to the occurrence of tuberculosis.

Dr. Hobby was also an assistant research clinical professor in public health at Cornell Medical College before retirement in 1977. In addition, she studied other subjects such as bacteriophage of *C. diphtheriae*, bacterial variation and enzymes, streptococci, pneumococci, rat-bite fever, rheumatic diseases, sulfonamides, immunizing agents, and germ-free life.

Dr. Hobby's number of publications has been tremendous. She authored more than 200 articles and made contributions to six books. She prepared the chapter titled "The Mode of Action of Streptomycin" in *Streptomycin*, edited by S. A. Waksman (1888–1976) in 1949, as well as a chapter titled "Terramycin" in *Therapeutics in Internal Medicine* in 1950. In 1954 she contributed a section titled "Synergism, Antagonism and Hormesis" in *Antibiotic Therapy*, edited by W. H. Welch (1850–1934). In 1960 she wrote a section titled "Antibiotics" in *Encyclopedia of Science and Technology* and an article titled "Viomycin" in the same book. In 1963 she contributed the chapter "Antimicrobial Susceptibility Tests" in *Diagnostic Procedures and Reagents*, fourth edition.

Dr. Hobby contributed to many professional organizations. She served as a member of the editorial boards of *Applied Microbiology* (1952–1958), *American Review of Respiratory Diseases* (1965–1968), and *Journal of Infectious Diseases* (1965–1972). She was the founder and editor of *Antimicrobial and Chemotherapy* (1965–1977). From 1962 to 1966, she represented the Veterans Administration on a study section of the National Institute of Allergy and Infectious Diseases, National Institutes of Health, Bethesda, Maryland. She was president of the New York Lung Association (1963–1965), vice president of the New York Trudeau Society (1966–1967), and vice president and chairman of the Long Range Planning Committee of the American Thoracic Society from 1968 to 1969. She served for many years as chair of the Laboratory Committee of the Veterans Administration Cooperative Study of Chemotherapy of Tuberculosis, and from 1972 to 1979 she was vice president and member of the Executive Committee of the International Society of Chemotherapy.

Dr. Hobby was also a member of many societies including the American Academy of Microbiology (charter fellow), the New York Academy of Sciences (fellow), the American Public Health Association (fellow), and the American Association for the Advancement of Science. She was an associate fellow of the New York Academy of Medicine; honorary member of the American Society for Microbiology; honorary member of the American Thoracic Society; and emeritus member of various other scientific organizations. Additionally, Dr. Hobby was listed in major biographic references, such as *American Men and Women of Science* (since 1955), *Who's Who of American Women*, *World Who's Who of Women*, and others.

Dr. Hobby received numerous awards and recognitions for her lifetime contributions. In 1951, she received the Mademoiselle Award in Science and the same year received the Commercial Solvents Award in Antibiotics, for the team of investigators at Pfizer, who had discovered oxytetracycline. In 1977 she received from the New York Lung Association an honorary award for 20 years of outstanding service toward improving community health in the fight against tuberculosis and other lung diseases.

In addition to scientific research, Dr. Hobby was a Christian active in church work. She was a member of the Madison Avenue Presbyterian Church in New York City and served as a member of the Board of Trustees of the Church (1971–1977) and co-chairman of the church's endowment fund campaign (1974–1978).

Dr. Hobby traveled widely through the United States, Canada, Europe, the British Isles, Japan, and Central and South America. Some of the travel was for professional purposes, but she also enjoyed the pleasures of learning about different cultures of many countries.

After her retirement, Dr. Hobby became a freelance science writer and a consultant. In 1985 at the age of 75, Dr. Hobby published a book titled *Penicillin: Meeting the Challenge*, in which she described in detail the story of penicillin. There, she described the unprecedented display of cooperation between different parties when American drug companies, governmental agencies, private hospitals, and numerous individual scientists, physicians, and administrators joined together to make the production of penicillin possible during wartime.

* * *

Dr. Gladys Hobby exhibited great compassion for human beings as well as great passion for the cure of human maladies. Like many distinguished women scientists, she had never married. Her life was dedicated totally to the understanding and treatment of infectious diseases. Through her work we can live better. She died of a heart attack on July 4, 1993.

20

GERTRUDE BELLE ELION
(1918–1999)

Innovative Drug Developer

> *Don't let others discourage you or tell you that you can't do it. In my day I was told women didn't go into chemistry. I saw no reason why we couldn't. It's true it took seven years of various jobs, including a year in graduate school and two years of high school teaching before the shortage of men in civilian jobs gave me the opportunity to prove myself. But after that, I never looked back.* —Gertrude Belle Elion (1921–1999)

Cancer is a complex disease that is complicated by environmental, viral, and genetic factors. Looking for anti-cancer drugs has been a long and enduring job for scientists, industries, and government. Gertrude Belle Elion stands out as an extraordinary expert in cancer chemotherapy. Her research revolutionized both drug-making and medicine, which transformed childhood leukemia from a disease that was 100 percent fatal to an illness that 80 percent of its young patients survived. She was chiefly responsible for the drugs that make organ transplants possible. She helped to develop treatment for gout and herpes. She and her research group developed the first drug that attacks viruses and were also instrumental in the development of the drug azidothymidine (AZT) that was the first drug approved by the Food and Drug Administration to fight adult immunodeficiency syndrome (AIDS). In addition, she demonstrated the differences in nucleic acid metabolism between normal cells and cancer cells. Her research contributed greatly to the progress of chemotherapy, pharmacology, immunology, and biochemistry. She was, therefore, awarded with a Nobel Prize along with George H. Hitchings (1905–1998) and Sir James W. Black (1924–) in 1988. She was a human jewel.

Gertrude Elion was born on January 23, 1918, in New York City. Her father was Robert Elion, and her mother was Bertha Cohen. Robert Elion was a descendent from a line of rabbis tracing back to 700. Around 1900, at the age of 12, Robert Elion migrated from Lithuania to New York and worked his way through New York University Dental School. Bertha Cohen was also an immigrant, from a region of Russia that eventually became Poland. Bertha came to the U.S. at the age of 14 and became a seamstress. Although she did not receive any college education, she was a prodigious reader. They lived in a middle-class neighborhood in Manhattan. Robert's father (Gertrude's grandfather) was a learned scholar and had been a rabbi in Russia. He migrated to the United States and moved in with Gertrude and her family in 1921. He made a living as a watchmaker in New York. Gertrude spent hours with her grandfather and had a close and loving relationship with him. Gertrude had a younger brother called Herbert who was born in 1924.

After Gertrude had attended the local grammar school, the family moved to the Bronx. Gertrude was a very smart girl. She had learned to read early and advanced rapidly in school, skipping several grades. As a child, she was hoping to attend college.

After grammar school, Gertrude attended Walton High School, an all-girl school with an excellent reputation. (Rosalyn Yalow [1921–], another Nobel Prize winner, was also a Walton High School graduate.) At the age of 15, Gertrude attended Hunter College, then the women's division of City College of New York. Hunter College is a tuition-free school. Had it not been free, Gertrude would probably not have been able to attend college because her father was bankrupted by the stock market crash in 1929.

In 1933 Gertrude's grandfather died of stomach cancer, which strengthened her determination to study science — chemistry — as a major. She said, "That was the turning point. It was as though the signal was there, 'this is the disease you're going to have to work against.' I never really stopped thinking about anything else. It was that sudden."

Gertrude graduated in 1937 at the age of 19 with an A.B. degree in chemistry, *summa cum laude*. She applied to 15 graduate schools but was rejected because she was a woman. She also could not find a job because of gender discrimination during the Great Depression. She said, "I hadn't been aware that there were doors closed to me until I started knocking on them. I went to an all-girls school. There were 75 chemistry majors in that class, but most were going to teach it.... When I got out and they didn't want women in the laboratory, it was a shock.... It was the Depression and nobody was getting jobs. But I had taken that to mean nobody was getting jobs —[when I heard] 'You are qualified. But we've never had a woman in the laboratory before, and we think you'd be a distracting influence,' I almost fell apart," Gertrude recalled. She was also surprised that she didn't get angry, but she was very discouraged.

About this time, Gertrude had met the man of her dreams, Leonard

Canter, a brilliant student majoring in statistics at City College who later worked for Merrill Lynch. They fell in love and decided to get married after Leonard returned from studying abroad for a year. Unfortunately, Leonard died prematurely of acute bacterial endocarditis, a bacterial infection of the heart, in 1941.

Gertrude spent the next seven years working in different jobs. To learn a profession, she started by going to a secretarial school. After six weeks in the school, she got a job as a doctor's receptionist (called laboratory assistant) and as an instructor to teach biochemistry to nursing students at New York University. She stayed on this job for only three months and then got a position as a chemist at a small pharmaceutical company, the Denver Chemical Company, for a salary of $12 per week (some sources say $20 per week). She worked for the company for a year and a half and saved $450. One of the reasons that she left the company was that each morning the company president told an anti–Semitic joke.

The next thing Gertrude did was to work again as a doctor's receptionist, working half-days to pay for carfare and lunch. She also took an education class on the side and became a substitute chemistry and physics teacher in a New York City high school. At the same time she enrolled in the master's program at New York University. She did her graduate work nights and weekends and obtained a master's degree in chemistry in 1941.

In 1942 Gertrude quit substitute teaching and obtained a laboratory job for A&P Grocery Stores. She worked as a quality control chemist, testing pickle acidity, measuring mayonnaise color, and measuring sugar concentrations in preserves. Although she liked the job in the beginning and learned a good deal about instrumentation, this job had nothing to do with cancer research. She looked for a job elsewhere. After a year and a half, she secured a research position at Johnson and Johnson Laboratories in New Brunswick, New Jersey. In this position, she had the opportunity to become familiar with the therapeutic drug called sulfonamides and fortified her interest in chemotherapy. However, the company there was closed after only six months, and her job was terminated. She began job hunting again.

Gertrude had a big turning point in her life in 1944. She had an interview with Dr. George H. Hitchings, director of Burroughs Wellcome Laboratories (now called Glaxo-Wellcome) in Tuckahoe, north of New York City. She was accepted by Dr. Hitchings and started a research position with an annual salary of $2,600. She began her career as a chemist on June 15, 1944. She stayed at this company for 40 years and made a great contribution to science and medicine.

During the 1950s, Elion attempted to get a Ph.D. degree while working at Burroughs Wellcome. She attended Brooklyn Polytechnic Institute, which offered graduate classes in chemistry and biochemistry in the evening. However, the graduate program required that she give up her job to continue her graduate work. She decided to forgo her graduate education and remain with Burroughs Wellcome.

In 1944 very little was known about the genetic material nucleic acid and its structure. Oswald T. Avery (1877–1955) and his group at Rockefeller Institute in New York demonstrated that DNA was the genetic material of living organisms and could transform bacteria and give it new genetic characteristics. This was an exciting breakthrough to science, and many scientists including Hitchings were interested in studying DNA. Hitchings wished to test one nucleic acid for antithyroid activity. He intended to use different nucleic acids to antagonize a known nucleic acid. Gertrude became excited at the creation of new chemicals that have biological activities. She endeavored to synthesize chemical compounds, which have similar structure to the building block of nucleic acids. One of the compounds, 2,6-diaminopurine (2,6-DAP), was found to inhibit the synthesis of nucleic acids in cancer cells. Further testing at Sloan-Kettering Institute for Cancer Research confirmed her findings. The compound was found active against mouse leukemia. This drug was also found effective in humans. Unfortunately, 2,6-DAP has several unfavorable side effects.

With the illustration of the double helix structure of DNA by Drs. James D. Watson (1928–), Francis H. C. Crick (1916–2004), Maurice H. F. Wilkins (1916–2004), and Rosalind Franklin (1920–1958), the interest in nucleic acid became the mainstream of research. Many enzymes for the biosynthesis of nucleic acids were isolated and described. Protein synthesis was also further elucidated. Gertrude became one of the forefront scientists involved in nucleic acid research. She continued to synthesize nucleic acid derivatives. Another compound she synthesized that turned out to be very useful was 6-mercaptopurine (6-MP), which was found to be effective in treating sarcoma in mice. This drug is marketed as Purinethol and in combination with other drugs is also useful in treating children with leukemia. This drug was approved by the FDA in 1953 as a viable treatment for acute childhood leukemia. This drug is still in use as a remission-inducing agent for maintenance therapy. Gertrude also synthesized thioguanine, another drug to be used in the treatment of leukemia in adults.

With the success of these drugs, Gertrude continued to synthesize a variety of derivatives of 6-MP and studied the metabolism and functions of these drugs *in vivo*. Her rationale was, "We have to understand the function of these drugs inside the body in order to truly cure diseases." Gertrude approached the research of 6-MP metabolism in the body using radioactive techniques. In 1958 researchers at Tuft University in Boston tested the immunosuppressive activities of azathioprine and thiamiprine, the derivatives of 6-MP, and found that azathioprine (trade name Imuran) could inhibit antibody-forming cells in rabbits. At this time, Dr. Roy Calne (1930–) and Joseph E. Murray (1919–) of Cambridge, England, requested a sample from Gertrude and tested the effect of azathioprine in dogs that received kidney transplants. They found that the production of rejecting antibodies was dramatically curtailed. In 1962 azathioprine was used for the first time in humans. Since then azathioprine has been used as the major antirejection drug for use in kidney transplant recipients.

During studies of 6-MP, Gertrude discovered that 6-MP would be broken down to thiouric acid by xanthine oxidase. She later discovered that allopurinol, another drug, could inhibit the activity of xanthine oxidase. Allopurinol could increase the immunosuppressive activity of 6-MP sevenfold by permitting the drug to remain in the tissue longer and also preventing the buildup of thiouric acid, which is toxic. In collaboration with researchers at Duke University, Gertrude discovered that allopurinol could treat a physiological disorder called gout. Patients with gout experience an accumulation of uric acid crystals in joints. Gertrude found that allopurinol could reduce the amount of uric acid considerably. This research led to the approval by the FDA in 1966 of using allopurinol (trade name Zyloprim) for treating gout.

During the 1970s Drs. J. Joseph Marr (1938–) and Randolph L Berens (1943–) of St. Louis University found that allopurinol was effective against pathogenic species of the protozoan Leishmania, which causes a sandfly-transmitted disease called leishmaniasis. Leishmaniasis occurs in tropical regions, in particular South America, and can cause a severe skin disease as well as visceral disease in which the protozoan infects multiple internal organs of the abdomen. Allopurinol was also effective against another South American problem, Chagas's disease, caused by protozoan *Trypanosoma cruzi* transmitted by an insect called the "kissing" bug. The bug lives in cracks of walls or in the roofing materials used in houses in South America. It comes out at night and bites people while they sleep. Chaga's disease can trigger autoimmunities and death by the age of thirty. Gertrude and her group discovered that allopurinol was converted to a certain toxic compound in the protozoan but not in animals or humans.

In 1968, the Burroughs Wellcome Laboratories were moved from Tuckahoe, New York, to Research Triangle Park, North Carolina. Elion eventually became an adjunct professor at Duke and the University of North Carolina, while continuing her research.

In the same year adenine arabinoside was reported to be antiviral, which intrigued Elion because of her previous work with the antiviral potential 2,6-DAP, which had a strong antiviral property but was very toxic to human cells. When Elion heard that arabinoside was antiviral, she immediately synthesized DAP-arabinoside and found that DAP-arabinoside was very inhibitory against DNA viruses including both varicella zoster, which causes shingles, and herpes simplex, which causes mouth and genital sores. Herpes infections can be fatal for patients with leukemia, cancer, and transplanted organs and marrow. Elion and her team studied DAP-arabinoside and related derivatives. With the help of Howard Schaeffer (1927–), the head of Burroughs Wellcome's organic chemistry division, and Lilia Beauchamp, the team further synthesized and modified the compounds and found that one derivative, acyclovir (acycloguanosine, trade name Zovirax), was an extremely good drug, preventing the replication of herpes viruses without toxic effects on the body. Besides treating shingles, acyclovir was also effective against Epstein-Barr virus, pseudo-rabies in animals, and herpes encephalitis, a frequently fatal brain infection in children. It is also effective for treating genital herpes.

Elion called acyclovir her final jewel. She said, "After that, everybody went to work in the field, so in addition to being an important compound, it was an important landmark." In 1982 acyclovir was approved by the FDA to be used in ointment and intravenous formulations and several years later in oral form. It is Burroughs Wellcome's largest-selling product, with worldwide sales of $838 million in 1991. Today, this drug is widely used for relieving the symptoms and pain of mouth and genital sores, chicken pox, and shingles.

Burroughs Wellcome allowed scientists to publish their findings after patents had been secured. Elion published more than 225 research papers throughout her career and many of those were her innovations. She was by all means a creative and productive scientific researcher.

Elion retired in 1983 and worked as a consultant. Her former unit, with the support of her expertise, continued to develop AZT, a drug effective against human immunodeficiency virus (HIV). The mechanism of action of AZT against HIV works in much the same way as acyclovir against the herpes viruses. AZT was approved by the FDA in 1987.

The American Chemical Society (ACS) awarded Elion its Garvan Medal in 1968. This was the only award that the ACS gave to a woman before 1980. She also received the President's Medal from Hunter College in 1970 and the Judd Award of the Sloan-Kettering Institute in 1983. In 1984 she won the Cain Award from the American Association for Cancer Research. In 1985 she received the Distinguished Chemist Award, and in 1990 she received the Ernst

W. Bertner Memorial Award from the M.D. Anderson Cancer Center and the Medal Honor from the American Cancer Society. In 1991 she received the National Medal of Science and was the first woman inducted into the Inventors Hall of Fame and the National Women's Hall of Fame. In 1997 she was awarded the Lemelson/MIT Lifetime Achievement Award.

Elion received a total of 25 honorary doctorates including those from Brown University, the University of Michigan, George Washington University, Hunter College of the City of New York, Philadelphia College of Pharmacy and Science, and Rensselaer Polytechnic Institute.

Elion also served as president of the American Association for Cancer Research (1983–1984) and on the National Cancer Advisory Board. She was elected to membership in the National Academy of Sciences in 1990 (and served on the council) and to the Institute of Medicine in 1991. She was a fellow of the American Academy of Pharmaceutical Scientists and the American Academy of Arts and Sciences; a foreign member of the Royal Society of Chemistry, the Transplantation Society, and an honorary member of the Spanish Academy of Dermatology and Venereology. She was on the World Health Organization (WHO) committees on three tropical diseases, filariasis, river blindness, and malaria. She served on the national committee for reviewing procedures for the approval of new cancer and AIDS drugs. She also served on the advisory committees for the American Cancer Society, the Leukemia Society of America, the board of the National Cancer Institute, the American Cancer Society, and the Multiple Sclerosis Society.

Elion worked with George H. Hitchings most of her life. Since Hitchings and Elion had written papers together for so long and had been considered a team, it is difficult to identify their respective contributions. In the laboratory, she was called "Trudy" and got along well with everybody. She was a senior research chemist from 1944 to 1963 and an assistant to director of the Division of Chemotherapy 1963 to 1967. Hitchings was always the boss, and he used "I" for their work while Elion used "we." When Hitchings retired from active research in 1967 to become vice president of research, Elion became head of the Department of Experimental Therapy and had the opportunity to show what she could do on her own. There was an undercurrent of competition between the two. Elvira Falco (1918–), a friend of both Hitchings and Elion for decades, said, "They worked together as well as any two people worked together. But I have a feeling that when your assistant gets as much credit as you have, it may be a difficult thing."

Elion's goal in research was to find new medicines to treat medically important challenges that weren't met at the time. She didn't do science in the abstract. She did it for a purpose, to advance a compound that might be useful to treat a disease. She tried to find the crucial experiment or series of experiments that would decide a question. Thomas Krenitsky (1938–), vice president of Burroughs Wellcome, said, "She's always herself. She's always Trudy. That guy (Hitchings) wasn't always the same person with everybody, but she is, whether the other person is a student, a glassware washer, or the president of the company. She's egalitarian, and she lives it. She's not elitist. That's for sure." He also further commented that she had real social conscience. "In fifty years, Trudy will have done more cumulatively for the human conditions than Mother Teresa." In 1989 when Burroughs Wellcome gave Hitchings and Elion $250,000 each to donate to charity, Elion gave hers to her alma mater for women's fellowships in chemistry and biochemistry.

Elion was a modest human being. She was often credited with the AZT development, because her former research group used her approach to produce the drug. But she declined the credit. She said, "The only thing I can claim is training people in the methodology.... The work is all theirs."

Besides working, Elion's favorite pastimes were opera, music, travel, and photography. She enjoyed music of Puccini, Verdi, and Mozart operas. Even after living in Research Triangle Park for years, she still flew to New York as often as possible for the Metropolitan Opera. She attended every classical musical concert, James Bond movie, and many of the college basketball games in the Research Triangle area. She enjoyed traveling. The reason she became interested in traveling was partly because her family seldom went away for vacation, and she was curious about the rest of the world. She had a close friend in her neighbor, Cora Himadi; together they traveled fairly widely over the world including Europe, Asia, Africa, and South America. Her interest in photography was also immense. She would do anything for a photograph including tramping up and down a mountain.

After retirement, she didn't stop working. She actually worked as hard as ever. She was interested in nurturing younger generations. She made herself readily accessible to graduate and medical students and freely gave her time to ensure that young people interested in science retained and developed that interest. She loved working and her enthusiasm for work was contagious. She said, "I don't want to die until I'm used up." On February 21, 1999, when she went for her daily walk, she collapsed and was taken to the University of North Carolina Hospital in Chapel Hill, where she died at midnight.

*   *   *

From the age of 15, Elion wanted to do cancer research, and she ultimately became one of most accomplished cancer researchers in the world. She was an employee of a pharmaceutical firm, her work was applied research, she had no Ph.D., and she was a woman, yet her accomplishments were extraordinary and amazed the world and the human race. She was involved directly with the development of at least five important drugs: thioguanine and mercaptopurine for the treatment of leukemia; azathioprine, an agent to prevent the rejection of kidney transplant and to treat rheumatoid arthritis; allopurinol for the treatment of gout; and acyclovir, the first selective antiviral agent that was effective against herpes virus infections. Her discoveries were not accidental, but came about by good planning. She developed drugs based on the understanding of basic biochemical and physiological processes and the differences in metabolism between normal cells and disease-causing cancer cells, protozoa, bacteria, and viruses. Studies of the metabolic differences of chemicals in different species are still the mainstream of research to biochemists, pharmacologists, and toxicologists.

Through it all, her friends said that Trudy was still Trudy. She was poised, unpretentious and as intent on curing diseases as she was when she dedicated her research to her grandfather, her mother, her fiancé, and the children with leukemia. Her favorite accolades were letters from patients and their relatives who benefited from her discovery. Elion is indeed a human jewel.

Further Reading

Alcamo, I. E. 1997. Gertrude Belle Elion (1918–). In *Women in the Biological Sciences: A Bio-bibliographic Sourcebook*. Edited by Louise S. Grinstein, Carol A. Biermann, and Rose K. Rose. Westport CT: Greenwood. 143–149.

Oakes, Elizabeth H., ed. 2002. Gertrude Belle ("Trudy") Elion. In *International Encyclopedia of Women Scientists*. New York: Facts on File. 102–103.

McGrayne, S. B. 1993. *Nobel Prize Women in Science: Their Lives, Struggles and Momentous Discoveries*. 2nd ed. Washington DC: Joseph Henry. 281–303.

Parrish, M. M. 1997. Gertrude Belle Elion. In *Notable Women in the Physical Sciences*. Edited by Benjamin F. Shearer and Barbara S. Shearer. Westport CT: Greenwood. 84–88.

21

JANE C. WRIGHT
(1919[?]–)

Pioneer of Cancer Chemotherapy

There's lots of fun in exploring the unknown. There's no greater thrill than in having an experiment turn out in such a way that you make a positive contribution.—Jane Cooke Wright (1919–)

Jane was born in late November of either 1919 or 1920.* She was born into a distinguished medical family. Her grandfather, Dr. Ceah Wright, was in 1881 one of the first graduates of Meharry Medical College in Nashville, Tennessee. After Dr. Ceah Wright died in 1895, her grandmother Lula Wright in 1899 married Dr. William Fletter Penn, who was the first African American to earn the M.D. degree from Yale Medical School. Dr. Penn's son-in-law, Dr. Harold D. West (1904–1974), was the first African American president of Meharry Medical College.

Jane's father was Dr. Louis Tompkins Wright (1891–1952), a well known surgeon, who graduated from Harvard Medical School and was the first African American to become a New York City police surgeon and to be appointed to the staff of a New York City hospital. As befits a police surgeon, Louis Wright pioneered developments in the treatment of gunshot and knife wounds, but he also developed an effective treatment for a sexually transmitted viral disease. He was the first to use a neck brace that allowed accident victims to be moved without risking permanent injuries to their spinal cords. Furthermore, he developed an internal splint that prevented permanent physical impairment in multiple breaks of major bones. At a time when there were no effective drugs for the treatment of cancer patients, Dr. Louis Wright was an innovator in the use of chemicals in the therapy of cancer. He also estab-

---

*Sources differ. Wright's birth date is reported to be November 20, 1920, by Distinguished African American Scientists of the 20th Century, and November 20, 1919, by Notable Black American Women; others reported it to be either November 17 or November 30, 1919.

lished the Cancer Research Foundation at Harlem Hospital in New York City. Jane's mother was Corinne Cooke Wright. Jane had a younger sister, Barbara, who also became a physician.

Jane Wright grew up in New York City in the family residence on 139th Street in the section of Manhattan known as Harlem, which was an upper-middle class neighborhood in the 1920s and 1930s. Jane attended exclusive private schools. The elementary school was called Ethical Culture School, and the high school was Fieldston Upper School. Jane did well in course work and was captain of the swimming team at Fieldston. She was awarded a four year scholarship to study art at Smith College in Northampton, Massachusetts. She was very interested in painting and considered becoming a professional artist, but her father discouraged this choice because of the financial uncertainty of a career in art. Since she was an excellent student, she changed her major from art to pre-medicine at the beginning of her third year in college. She graduated with a B.A. in 1942 and was admitted to New York Medical School the same year.

In 1942 the United States was deeply involved in World War II, which led to many changes in college life. Due to the shortage of doctors for the military service, medical training was shortened from four to three years with the addition of training during the summer months. Jane did very well in medical school. She was vice-president of her class, president of the honor society, and literary editor of the yearbook. While the compressed program was grueling, Jane was able to graduate with honors in June of 1945, third in a class of ninety-five. Right after her graduation, she was an intern at Bellevue Hospital in New York City (1945–1946). In 1946 she became assistant resident. Her supervisor at Bellevue called her "by all odds the most promising intern I have ever had working with me."

From 1947 to 1948, Jane did her residency practice in internal medicine at Harlem Hospital. Jane initially planned to enter private practice in general medicine, but her father had just established the Cancer Research Foundation at Harlem Hospital and invited his daughter to collaborate with him on his research program. So Jane worked as visiting physician at Harlem Hospital in addition to her employment as a New York City school physician. Later that year, she became a clinician at the Cancer Research Foundation at Harlem Hospital and devoted her study to the effects of drugs on tumors and other abnormal growths.

Jane Wright's interest in chemotherapy for cancer patients was inspired by her father. During World War I, Dr. Louis Wright served as a first lieutenant in the Medical Corps in France, where he suffered permanent lung damage from a poisonous gas attack. In 1942 a ship carried soldiers and a quantity of the chemical weapon nitrogen mustard gas to Europe. When the ship sank in the Italian port of Bari, many soldiers were killed by the escaped poison gas. From this incident, medical doctors noticed that the gas reduced the number of white blood cells of the victims. White blood cells are the first line of defense against bacterial or viral infection in normal, healthy persons. But in leukemia patients, there is overproduction of white blood cells. Since mustard gas can reduce the number of white blood cells, medical doctors thought that a chemical like mustard gas might kill cancerous white blood cells and cure leukemia.

Having had personal experience with poison gas attacks and considering what had been learned about the effect of mustard gas, Dr. Louis Wright became interested in chemotherapy for cancer patients. He thought that there must be some chemicals that could cure cancer. Louis and his daughter worked as a team, studying drugs and trying a variety of possible cancer treatments. When Dr. Louis Wright died of a heart attack in 1952, Dr. Jane Wright became director of the Cancer Research Foundation and continued to diligently and tirelessly work as if it were a special call for her life.

In September 1955 Jane became director of cancer chemotherapy research and instructor of research surgery in the department of surgery of the New York University Medical Center. Within five months, she was appointed assistant professor, and in 1961 she was adjunct professor of research surgery. Dr. Jane Wright taught classes in surgical research and pursued her studies of cancer fighting chemicals at both Harlem Hospital and the New York University Medical Center. Her work in analyzing the efficacy of a wide range of drugs in the treatment of cancer produced a better understanding of the relationships of response to a drug in patients, tissue cultures, or animals. She stressed that responses to the same drug may be different in research animals and in human beings as well as in the patient and in cultured cells of his very own cancer.

One of the unique contributions of Dr. Wright was the use of mithramycin in cancer therapy. She thought that this drug could be used against a type of brain tumor found deeply hidden in the brain and almost impossible to remove by surgery. She and her team tested the drug on fourteen patients who were near death. Eight of them improved and three out of the eight were totally cured. She postulated that given the right drugs, cure is always possible.

In 1961 Dr. Jane Wright was invited to join a team of physicians to tour Kenya and what is now Tanzania under the sponsorship of the African Research Foundation. They traveled in a mobile medical unit through the African countryside and introduced modern medical services to people who were not aware of the availability of modern medicine. Although the journey lasted only three weeks, Dr. Jane Wright developed a strong interest in helping African people and later became a vice president of the African Research Foundation.

In 1964 she was called by the White House to be a member of the Presidential Commission on Heart Disease, Cancer, and Stroke. The report of this commission led to the establishment of a network of research centers across the country. This network helped facilitate the communication between different research laboratories.

In July of 1967 Dr. Jane Wright returned to her alma mater, New York Medical College, as a professor of surgery and associate dean, which was the highest position for an African American woman in a major medical school at that time. She also joined the staff of its affiliated hospitals, Flower-Fifth Avenue, Metropolitan, and Bird S. Coler Memorial. She became an administrator of the medical school and was personally responsible for the development of a program to study cancer, heart disease, and stroke.

In addition to her administrative duties, Dr. Jane Wright actively pursued her cancer research. Since different cancers respond differently to the same drug — and the same cancer might respond differently in two different patients — she developed a tissue culture technique to test the effect of a given anticancer drug on a patient's very own cancer cells. The reasoning was that if the drug was effective in killing the person's cancer cells in the tissue culture, then that drug had a high chance of being effective. She also experimented with techniques for injecting anticancer drugs directly into the location of the cancer rather than into a more conveniently exposed vein or artery. She also developed surgical ways of temporarily rerouting arteries that fed the site of the cancer. The anticancer drug would go to the location of the tumor and nowhere else in the patient's body, thus minimizing the negative side effects of the drug. She also pioneered giving her patients combinations of drugs at the same time. She aggressively treated persistent cancers using all the medical weapons available including surgery, radiation, and chemicals. Dr. Jane Wright continued to concentrate on and develop new ideas for cancer therapy. She and her father led the fight against cancer by developing techniques and treatments that have saved or prolonged the lives of many cancer patients. She published numerous research articles related to cancer therapy that were translated, abstracted, and quoted all over the world.

Dr. Jane Wright received numerous honors and awards. The first notable award was the Merit Award from Mademoiselle in 1952. In 1965 she received the Spirit of Achievement Award of the Women's Division of the Albert Einstein College of Medicine for her deep commitment as scientist and teacher in advancing medical knowledge and research. In 1967 she was bestowed with the Hadassah Myrtle Wreath Award for the outstanding contribution she made to her field. In 1968 Smith College presented her with the Smith Medal. The December issue of *Cancer Research* in 1975 saluted eight senior women scientists in observance of the International Women's Year. Dr. Jane Wright was included among them.

In 1965 Dr. Jane Wright received an honorary degree from Women's Medical College (now the Medical College of Pennsylvania). She received another from Denison University in 1971.

She was elected to the Alpha Omega Alpha National Honorary Medical Society in 1966. She served on the board of trustees of Smith College and of the New York City Division of the American Cancer Society. She also served as vice-president of the African Research Foundation and was on the editorial board of the *Journal of the National Medical Association*. In addition, she was a member of numerous professional organizations and was cited by many civic groups for her outstanding contributions.

In 1983 Dr. Jane Wright was invited to give a presentation of her work at the annual convention of the National Medical Association. In her presentation, "Cancer Therapy: Past, Present, and Future," she covered the historical milestones in the development of chemical control of cancer, including her own work. This speech resulted in a multipart series of review articles entitled "Update in Cancer Chemotherapy," which were published in the *Journal of the National Medical Association* beginning in 1984.

Dr. Jane Wright was a devoted scientist and a very highly regarded administrator. She was also a great human being. She married David Jones, Jr., on July 27, 1947. David Jones was a Harvard Law School graduate and son of Bennett College president Dr. David D. Jones. They had two daughters, Jane and Alison. Away from her job at the medical school, she was known as Mrs. David Jones or simply Jane Jones. Mr. Jones was an attorney and later became prominent as a founder of anti-poverty and job training organizations for young African Americans. These were causes that Jane sincerely supported. In 1952 when she received the Merit Award from Mademoiselle, she was quoted in the journal *Crisis* as saying, "My plans for the future are to continue seeking a cure for cancer, to be a good mother to my children, and a good wife to my husband." Unfortunately, her husband died of heart failure in 1976. Dr. Jane Wright retired officially in 1987. She was eventually named professor emeritus of New York Medical College. Besides, scientific work, she enjoyed watercolor painting, reading mysteries, and sailing.

*   *   *

Dr. Jane Wright was not only very capable but also very fortunate. Somehow she managed to escape many of the effects of the gender and race discrimination common in her era. Her father, who did have to constantly fight against racial injustice — he held the American Medical Association responsible for racial discrimination in medical care and publicly stated that "the American Medical Association has demonstrated as much interest in the health of the Negro as Hitler has in the health of the Jew" — blazed the trail for her. She was given good opportunities in every respect, went smoothly all the way from grade school to medical doctor, and held many good positions. Nevertheless, without her genuine hard work, she would not have made such a significant contribution. It was her tireless effort, coupled with her knowledge and technique, that brought her to the light of success. In addition, she must have had a charisma that helped her to win the support of so many people in her life. Dr. Jane Wright was by all means a distinguished woman scientist.

Further Reading

American Men and Women of Science. 1983. 16th ed. Vol. 8. New York: Bowker.

Cazort, J. E. 1992. Jane C. Wright. In *Notable Black American Women.* Edited by Jessie Carney Smith. Vol. 2. Detroit: Gale Research. 1283–1285.

Crisis **60** (January 1953): 4–5.

Current Biography. 1968. New York: Wilson.

Kessler, J. H., J. S. Kidd, R. A. Kidd, and K. A. Morin. 1996. *Distinguished African American Scientists of the Twentieth Century.* Phoenix AZ: Oryx. 350–353.

Medical family. *Ebony* **6** (January 1951): 71–74.

Warren, Wini. 1999. *Black Women Scientists in the United States.* Bloomington: Indiana University Press. 277–284.

Who's Who in America. 1989. 45th ed. Vol. 2. Wilmette IL: Marquis.

22

ROSALIND ELSIE FRANKLIN
(1920–1958)

Critical Figure in Determining the
Double Helix Structure of DNA

Many female scientists have worked just as hard and accomplished just as much as their male counterparts without receiving equal recognition. Even though they participated in the most cutting-edge research and their work was undoubtedly first class, their names were often left out when rewards were considered. Rosalind Franklin was one such scientist.

Rosalind E. Franklin made important contributions to the understanding of cellular structures. Furthermore, she provided the scientific evidence of X-ray crystallography of deoxyribonucleic acid (DNA), which was used by James Watson (1928–), Francis Crick (1916–2004), and Maurice Wilkins (1916–2004) for the determination of their double-helix structure. These three men received the Nobel Prize in 1962 for their illustration of the DNA structure. None of their three Nobel lectures cited Franklin's work. However, Wilkins did mention her in his acknowledgments.

Rosalind was born on July 25, 1920, in London. Her father was Ellis Franklin, and her mother was Muriel Waley Franklin. Ellis was a professor at the Working Men's College in London, and he also worked in a merchant bank. Ellis Franklin's grandfather, Abraham Franklin, was the first member of the Franklin family to go to England. They came from Breslau, Germany, and settled in London in 1763. Abraham Franklin established himself as a merchant banker and prospered in his career. Muriel was the daughter of Jacob Cohen, who was a professor of political economy at the University College, London. Rosalind was the second of five children and the first daughter. The family was wealthy and highly educated. Ellis Franklin assumed that his Rosalind would follow the family tradition, which was to concentrate their efforts on helping the disadvantaged members of the community and taking their rightful place in society. Rosalind's parents did not encourage her to pursue an independent career.

Rosalind attended St. Paul's Girls' School, which was one of the few schools that taught science courses to female students in those days. Rosalind was very good in physics and chemistry and was awarded a foundation scholarship at the school. At age 15 she decided to pursue a career in science. She graduated from St. Paul in 1938 and then went to Paris to study French for a while. In the same year, she enrolled at Newnham College in Cambridge, London, and obtained her B.S. degree in 1941 with high honors. Immediately following graduation, she was offered a research scholarship at Newnham to pursue graduate studies. She studied gas-phase chromatography with Dr. Ronald G. W. Norrish (1897–1978) for a year. However, she found Dr. Norrish difficult to work with. Consequently, she accepted a position as an assistant research officer with the British Coal Utilization Research Association (CURA).

At CURA Rosalind did research on the microstructures of coals. She applied the knowledge of physical chemistry that she had learned in college to her study of coals. From 1942 to 1946 she published five research papers, three of them were authored by her alone. She submitted her dissertation, *The Physical Chemistry of Solid Organic Colloids with Special Relation to Coal and Solid Materials*, to Cambridge and obtained her Ph.D. in 1945. In 1946 Rosalind attended a conference on carbon research in London and presented a paper. During the conference, she met Dr. Marcel Mathieu, a distinguished scientist from France. Dr. Mathieu was responsible for a great part of French scientific research. Dr. Mathieu recognized Rosalind's scientific ability and offered her a position as "Chercheur" at the Laboratoire Central des Service Chimique de L'Etat. Rosalind accepted the position and moved to Paris in February of 1947. At the Laboratoire, Rosalind learned the technique of X-ray diffraction. Applying the technique, she was able to describe the structure of carbon and the changes that occur when carbon is heated to form graphite. This technique allowed her later to study the structure of DNA.

In Paris she became fluent in French under the tutelage of Jacques Mehring, one of the leading scientists in Paris. She was hard-working, sociable, and easygoing with her colleagues. According to Vittorio Luzzati, a colleague of Rosalind's, and to a recent book, *Rosalind Franklin: The Dark Lady of DNA*, by Brenda Maddox, Rosalind enjoyed lunch discussions on politics, philosophy, and human rights with her colleagues. She also enjoyed swimming, hiking, and mountaineering. She dressed stylishly for important occasions and adopted the fashionable New Look of 1947. This might have been the most happy and rewarding period of Rosalind's life, according to her close friend Anne Piper. She got along well with her colleagues, and her contributions were appreciated. She did not experience any sexual discrimination.

Because of her citizenship, her employment at the laboratory in Paris was not permanent. She had to find a job elsewhere. Dr. John Randall (1905–1984) at the Medical Research Council at King's College, London, was interested in applying X-ray diffraction skills to the study of DNA structure. He offered Rosalind the Turner Newall Research Fellowship to encourage her coming to work for him. This was a hard decision for her since she enjoyed life in Paris. Rosalind sought the advice of Dorothy Hodgkin, a distinguished British chemist who was awarded a Nobel Prize for her work on the determination of vitamin B_{12} using X-ray crystallography in 1964. Dr. Hodgkin encouraged her to go back to England. Dr. Randall also promised that she would be working on one of the more pressing research problems of the time: puzzling out the structure of DNA. Rosalind accepted the fellowship in 1951. Shortly after starting to work in Dr. Randall's laboratory, Rosalind was charged with the task of setting up an X-ray diffraction unit in the laboratory to produce diffraction pictures of DNA. Rosalind worked closely with a student, Mr. Raymond Gosling, who had been attempting to capture pictures of the elusive DNA.

However, another scientist, Dr. Maurice Wilkins, was already working in the laboratory on the same problem as Rosalind. Dr. Randall did not inform Dr. Wilkins that Rosalind's assignment was to take charge of the X-ray laboratory to investigate the structure of DNA. Dr. Wilkins thought that Dr. Franklin was hired as his assistant since Dr. Wilkins was the second man in command next to Dr. Randall in the laboratory. This was further complicated by the poor arrangement when Rosalind arrived at the laboratory. When Rosalind first reported to work, Dr. Wilkins was on vacation. When Dr. Wilkins returned from vacation, he discovered that his laboratory was occupied and rearranged by Dr. Franklin. Furthermore, Mr. Raymond Gosling was no longer working for Dr. Wilkins but for Rosalind. This certainly created a great discomfort for Dr. Wilkins. Dr. Wilkins showed a dislike for her the first time they met. Anne Sayre, a biographer, suggested that the discomfort might also have come from the fact that Dr. Wilkins was slightly older than Rosalind and expected more respect because of seniority. However, Rosalind had a strong personality and expected to be equal in everything. She made no apology for the fact that she was a woman. Or there could have been professional jealousy, which so commonly occurred with those who were working on the same project.

Dr. Wilkins and Rosalind's mutual dislike was made worse by the fact that women were not allowed to lunch in the Senior Common Room. Rosalind's male colleagues could include ex-military men who had a tough, ferocious approach that spilled over into beer-drinking camaraderie. They were not used to treating women as their peers. Rosalind did not accept their discriminatory behavior. Gentle deference was not her style. Because of her educational and family background, she expected to be treated politely. Determined to stand her ground, she refused to be browbeaten and would become combative under pressure. Her aggressive intelligence could also be stung into defending territory that she saw as her own by means of vicious attack. This part of her character was shown when she worked in the environment where sexual prejudice prevailed.

There was still animosity between Rosalind and Wilkins, despite common ground such as the fact that both of them had studied at Cambridge and both of them had worked overseas. They could communicate amicably about theater, books, and politics, but they never discussed science. Wilkins considered Rosalind peremptory, off-handed, and spiky. Historian Paul Strathern pointed out in his book *Crick, Watson and DNA* that the irritable relationship between Wilkins and Rosalind was due to their temperaments as well as to the social climate of the day. Dr. Wilkins was soft spoken, deliberative, and shy; Rosalind was single-minded, articulate, determined, competitive, argumentative, and passionate. The chemistry between the two was strongly negative.

Despite their dislike and distrust for each other, they pursued their research diligently and effectively. For instance, Rosalind X-rayed DNA fibers that Wilkins had obtained from a Swiss investigator. A few months after joining the laboratory, Rosalind was ready to make a presentation of her new findings. In November of 1951, Rosalind presented her findings of the discovery that DNA could exist either as A form (dry) or as B form (wet). According to her X-ray diffraction pictures, the DNA could transform from a crystalline A form to a B form with an increase in relative humidity. She also suggested that the phosphate groups might lie outside the molecule.

In Rosalind's audience that day was Dr. James Watson, who was working with Dr. Francis Crick at the Cavendish Laboratory in Cambridge under the directorship of Lawrence Bragg (1890–1971). Dr. Bragg and his team included eminent researchers Max Perutz (1914–2002) and John Kendrew (1917–1997). Drs. Watson and Crick were very interested in unraveling the molecular structure of DNA. They had once built a DNA structure model, but it was not a correct one. Dr. Franklin was invited to see the model they built and gave a serious criticism on the errors of the model. Drs. Crick and Watson invited Franklin to collaborate with them to do the DNA model building, but Dr. Franklin rejected their invitation. Dr. Bragg considered the model built by Drs. Crick and Watson an embarrassing failure. He ordered them to stop the model building of DNA and asked them to study something else. Dr. Watson disliked Rosalind — possibly from the first time he heard her speak — and now his dislike deepened.

In Rosalind's published reports, she suggested the probability that the B form of DNA exhibited the helical structure. She continued to study the A form, which produced a more readable X-ray photograph. But the A form does not show the double-helical structure as clearly as the B form. In late spring of 1952 Rosalind traveled to Yugoslavia to visit a coal research laboratory for a month. When she returned, she and her student, Gosling, continued to investigate the A form of DNA but found no new information. Rosalind also began to do model building but could not think of any structure that would accommodate all of the evidence she obtained from her X-ray diffraction pictures. She did rule out single or multi-stranded helical models. In her Medical Research Council (MRC) report, she also noticed the symmetrics of the double helix.

In late December of 1952 Dr. Watson learned from Dr. Peter Pauling, son of Linus Pauling (1901–1994), who was also interested in solving the structure of DNA, that Linus Pauling and Robert Corey (1897–1971) were about to solve the structure. In fact, they submitted a paper titled "A Proposed Structure for the Nucleic Acids" to the *Proceedings of the National Academy of Sciences*. Both Watson and Crick were downcast by the news. Dr. Watson told the news to Rosalind when she made her last presentation at the King's College since she had already decided to move to a laboratory that would offer a more friendly working environment. Dr. Watson perhaps told her that she could not solve the structure of DNA alone because Dr. Linus Pauling was going to solve the problem ahead of her. He might have implied that Rosalind lacked the mental ability to transfer the diffraction photographs into a structure. Their meeting resulted in a big argument. Dr. Watson said that she would have struck him if he had not left her office in time. Their relationship was down to the bottom.

It turned out that the DNA structure proposed by Drs. Pauling and Corey was erroneous because it was based on the X-ray photograph obtained by Dr. William T. Astbury (1898–1961). Dr. Astbury's X-ray photograph of DNA had been a combination of both A form and B form.

About this time Watson and Crick were busy in their construction of the DNA model. Dr. Watson could not get the hard crystallographic data from Rosalind. However, Dr. Wilkins, without Rosalind's knowledge, showed him the DNA diffraction pictures that Rosalind had amassed. (In May of 1952, someone gave a beautiful X-ray picture of DNA to Dr. Wilkins. Dr. Wilkins labeled the picture Photograph 51.) Watson saw the evidence he needed to prove the double helical structure of DNA and immediately returned to Crick in Cambridge. They put all the evidence together and figured the double helical structure of DNA. On February 28, 1953, they showed the model to Rosalind, and she immediately saw the accuracy of the DNA model. Drs. Crick and Watson quickly submitted the Nobel Prize winning paper, "Molecular Structure of Nucleic Acids: A Structure for Deoxyribose Nucleic Acid," to *Nature,* and it was published on April 25, 1953. In this paper, they did not acknowledge that the X-ray diffraction photograph was produced by Rosalind. This paper was followed, in the same issue of *Nature,* by another one by Wilkins, Stokes and Wilson titled "Molecular Structure of Deoxypentose Nucleic Acids," in which they interpreted their X-ray photograph in support of the Watson and Crick model.

Rosalind and Gosling had been working on a paper of their own. Rosalind had deduced the sugar-phosphate backbone of the helix before Watson and Crick's model was made public. She devoted her time to the study of the A form of the DNA crystallography, and thus missed the importance of the B form, which gives the true helical information of DNA. Rosalind and Gosling wrote a paper titled "Molecular Configuration in Sodium Thymonucleate" that was published in the same issue of *Nature* (April 1953). In *Nature's* July issue of the same year, Rosalind and Gosling published another important paper titled "Evidence for 2-chain Helix in the Crystalline Structure of Sodium Deoxyribonucleate," which provided essential evidence for the double-helix theory.

Drs. Watson and Crick not only utilized the X-ray photograph behind Rosalind's back, but they also convinced Dr. L. Bragg to lobby Dr. John Maddox, editor of *Nature,* to publish their paper first and commented that Rosalind's general idea was inconsistent with their model. In other words, they tried to minimize the contribution of Rosalind. In fact, Rosalind clearly indicated the symmetrical double helix nature of DNA in her MRC report dated February 14, 1953.

The Watson, Crick, and Wilkins paper in 1953 was the basis for the award of the Nobel Prize in 1962 because it explained correctly the double helix structure of DNA. Rosalind and Gosling's papers gave great insight into the structures of DNA, but as Francis Crick said, "Rosalind Franklin was only two steps away from the solution [of the structure]. She needed to realize that the two [sugar-phosphate] chains must run in opposite directions and that bases, in their correct tautomeric form, were paired together."

Dr. Watson's comments on Dr. Franklin had done a great deal of damage to her relationship with other people. She was pictured as a "dark lady." When she decided to move to Birkbeck College to work in the unit of Dr. J. D. Bernal (1901–1971), Dr. Randall made a clear statement that the DNA project was to stay in his laboratory. She could not continue her work on the DNA structure if she left. Although Gosling had been warned against further association with Rosalind, Gosling continued to seek Rosalind's advice in private and to finish their DNA research.

Rosalind seemed to enjoy working in Dr. Birkbeck's laboratory. There were a few things that were rather inconvenient by today's standards. For example, she worked in a small laboratory on the fifth floor while the X-ray equipment was in the basement. She had to trek up and down stairs because there was no elevator in the building. The roof leaked, and she had to set out pots and pans to catch the water. Sometime in 1956, Rosalind lost grant support from the Agricultural Research Council (ARC) because she had a severe argument with a man who was in charge of the agency. Rosalind bitterly complained. She said, "The ARC refused to support any project that had a woman directing it." Luckily, Rosalind successfully sought funding from the United States Public Health Service and kept her research actively going. Dr. Franklin endeavored to do a lot of work with a small amount of money.

In Dr. Birkbeck's laboratory, Rosalind devoted her major effort to uncovering the structure of the tobacco mosaic virus (TMV). She collaborated with Dr. Aaron Klug (1926–), a South African scientist, who joined the laboratory the year after Rosalind began in Dr. Birkbeck's laboratory. By 1956 she had obtained some of the best pictures ever made of the crystallographic structure of TMV and, with her colleagues, disproved the notion that TMV was the solid cylinder with RNA in the middle and a protein subunit on the outside. She showed that the cylinder was hollow and that the RNA lay embedded in the protein subunits. She also initiated work that supported the hypothesis that the RNA was single stranded. Her group was the world's leader in using X-ray diffraction to uncover the molecular structures of viruses. Her contribution to the knowledge of the structure of the RNA virus TMV was unparalleled.

In 1956 Rosalind visited several laboratories in the United States including the ones at California Institute of Technology, Washington University, Yale University, and the University of California, Berkeley. In Berkeley, she worked with Dr. Wendell Stanley (1904–1971) for about a month. There was a story that showed how her reputation was terribly damaged by Dr. Watson and others. On one occasion, there was a laboratory picnic party to which Drs. Crick, Wilkins, and Rosalind were all invited. However, Rosalind could not find a ride to the picnic because everyone had been warned by Dr. Watson about her supposedly unpleasant character. Dr. Stanley had to drive her to the party. Students and others found out that she was actually a very friendly and fun-loving person.

Upon returning to England in the fall, Rosalind became sick. She was diagnosed as having ovarian tumors, which were removed by surgery. The following year she had a second surgery. Even though she was in poor health, she began to work on the polio virus and did not stop working despite her sickness and pain. For a time, she kept a sample of crystallized polio virus in a thermos in her family's refrigerator. In 1957 the Brussels World's Fair Committee in Belgium requested that Rosalind build two models of virus molecules to display at the 1958 World's Fair. She and her group designed a model of tobacco mosaic virus for the occasion. But she did not live long enough to see her model displayed in Brussels. She died of cancer on April 16, 1958, at the age of 37. The six-foot model was moved to the new campus of Medical Research Council Laboratory of Molecular Biology outside of Cambridge.

Rosalind's death was a shock to the scientific community. Excess exposure to X-ray was certainly the ultimate reason for her contracting cancer.

In 1962, four years after the death of Rosalind, Watson, Crick, and Wilkins were awarded the Nobel Prize in Medicine or Physiology. Rosalind was not included because the Nobel Committee honors only living scientists. Had she lived until 1962, she should have shared the Nobel Prize.

Although Rosalind Franklin was not awarded the Nobel Prize, there is a blue plaque near her flat at the corner of the Fulham Road and Drayton Gardens on the wall at King's College in London. The plaque commemorated all those who were involved in the DNA work. The four names, including Rosalind's, are on the plaque.

* * *

Rosalind Franklin was excluded from the circle of those working on DNA structure because of numerous reasons that are beyond the analysis of this author. Her reputation had been seriously damaged by Dr. Watson. In his book *The Double Helix*, Watson characterized Rosalind as competitive, stubborn, and unfeminine. Dr. Watson believed that Franklin was not capable of transferring the diffraction photographs into a structure. However, this was not true at all. Rosalind's insight led to closer truth than Crick and Watson's first uninformed guess of the DNA structure in 1951. Rosalind was criticized by refusing to share the hard X-ray diffraction photographs for model building with Watson and Crick. However, Rosalind did freely share her X-ray photographs with Dr. Linus Pauling's collaborator, Robert Corey, who was also working on the DNA structure modeling.

Neither Dr. Francis Crick nor Dr. Max Perutz (1914–2002) approved of the insults to Rosalind and others in Watson's first draft of *The Double Helix*. Linus Pauling even tried to veto its publication. Dr. Watson changed his comments about Rosalind. He wrote, "Since my initial impressions of her, both scientific and personal, were often wrong, I want to say something here about her achievements. The X-ray work she did at King's is increasingly regarded as superb. The sorting out of A and B forms, by itself, would have made her reputation; even better was her 1952 demonstration using Patterson superposition methods, that the phosphate groups must be on the outside of the DNA molecule."

In reality Rosalind was a devoted, hard-working scientist who suffered from her colleagues' reluctance to treat her with respect because of her gender. Anne Sayre's biography, *Rosalind Franklin and DNA*, refuted in detail the criticisms of her in Watson's book *The Double Helix*. Others argued that Sayre's book was inaccurate. Maurice Wilkins believed that any scientific discovery was rarely the work of one person or a team. Instead, he thought that breakthroughs came via a series of conclusions, over a period of years, often with unconnected teams working on slightly related topics. Francis Crick also said, "It was more than just Kings and Cavendish, there were teams in Scandinavia and in the United States whose work was vital to ours." A scientific hypothesis often derives from the previous findings. Sometimes those findings are wrongly interpreted and later corrected to lead to the next better hypothesis. The model of DNA structure illustrated in the paper by Watson, Crick, and Wilkins in 1953 derived from several previous models that were inaccurate.

However, it is fair to say that there is no doubt about the contribution of Rosalind to the discovery of the structure of DNA.

Nonetheless, the life story of Rosalind is mixed with gender discrimination and professional jealousy. As Alexander Fleming (1881–1955) remarked, "Professional jealousy can be a most brutal and terrifying phenomenon." Gender bias and professional jealousy are still prevalent in the world today.

(This article was reproduced with the permission of *Society of Industry Microbiology News* 54:10–15, 2004.)

Further Reading

Bernal, J. D. 1958. Dr. Rosalind Franklin. *Nature* **182**: 154.

Franklin, R. E. 1951. Crystallite growth in graphitizing and nongraphitizing carbons. *Proceedings of the Royal Society* **209**A: 154.

Franklin, R. E., and A. Klug. 1958. Order-disorder transitions in structures containing helical molecules. *Discussions of the Faraday Society* **25**: 104–110.

Franklin, R. E., and R. G. Gosling. 1953. Evidence for 2-chain helix in crystalline structure of sodium deoxyribonucleate. *Nature* **172**: 156–157.

Klug, A. 1968. Rosalind Franklin and the discovery of the structure of DNA. *Nature* **219**: 808–810; 843–844.

Maddox, B. 2002. *Rosalind Franklin: The Dark Lady of DNA*. New York: HarperCollins.

The New Zealand edge: heroes: scientists: Maurice Wilkins. www.nzedge.com/heroes/
   wilkins.html
Piper, A. 1998. Rosalind Franklin: light on a dark lady. *Trends in Biochemical Science* **23**:
   151–154.
Sayre, A. 1975. *Rosalind Franklin and DNA*. New York: Norton.
Strathern, 1999. *Crick, Watson, and DNA*. Garden City NY: Doubleday.
Watson, James D. 1968. *The Double Helix*. New York: Atheneum.

23

ROSALYN SUSSMAN YALOW
(1921–)

Co-Developer of Radioimmunoassay Procedure

The trouble with discrimination is not discrimination per se, but rather that the people who are discriminated against think themselves as second class. There was something wrong with the discriminator, not something wrong with me.

I still think discovery is the most exciting thing in the world.—Rosalyn Sussman Yalow (1921–)

Rosalyn S. Yalow and Solomon A. Berson (1918–1972) developed the radioimmunoassay (RIA) procedure, which is a significant advancement in medicine and has found multiple applications. The procedure can detect minute changes in hormones, which can help diagnosis and treatment of numerous medical conditions, as in the case of children with dwarfism who are treated with human growth hormones, or newborns who are treated to prevent retardation caused by underactive thyroids. RIA is also used in blood banks to screen for deadly diseases. It helps infertile couples who are tested for insufficient sex hormones; fetuses who are checked for serious deformities like spina bifida; athletes who are tested for drug abuse; crime victims who are tested for poisons; and others.

The availability of RIA gave the new science of neuroendocrinology a quantum leap. Because of Yalow's contribution, in 1977 she was awarded the Nobel Prize in Medicine or Physiology, sharing it with Roger Guillemin (1924–) and Andrew V. Schally (1926–).

Rosalyn was born July 19, 1921, in the South Bronx of New York City. Her father was Simon Sussman, who was born on the Lower East Side of New York. Mr. Sussman had a paper and twine business. Her mother was Clara Zipper Sussman, who came from Germany at the age of four. Neither of her parents received a high school education. Rosalyn had an older brother called Alexander. Rosalyn learned to read before kindergarten. By the time she was

169

only five years old, she and her brother were making weekly trips to the local public library. In order to join the library, she learned to read the statement and signed her name as required by the library regulations. She was so good in her studies that she skipped a few grades in grammar school. She was very independent and persistent about what she wanted to do, and she would work for what she wanted. In New York, she attended Public School 51 and Public School 10. At the age of eight, she had decided to get married, have children, and be a noted scientist. "I liked knowing things. The thing I like is logic, and this characterizes all of science," she said. At the age of ten, she was enrolled in a girls' junior school. By the seventh grade she was devoted to mathematics. At that age she had already set her life goal: medical research. She completed three grades in two years and continued her studies at the famous Walton High School. (Getrude Elion [1918–1999], another Nobel Prize winner, attended that high school before her.) At Walton High School, a chemistry teacher, Mr. Mondzak, encouraged her interest in chemistry. She graduated from high school at the age of 15 and was admitted to Hunter College (now the City University of New York). (Getrude Elion also attended this college.)

At Hunter College, professors Herbert Otis and Duane Roller (1894–1965) inspired her interest in physics. In 1939 nuclear fission was discovered by Lise Meitner (1878–1968), Otto Hahn (1879–1968), and Fritz Strassman (1902–1980). About this time, Enrico Fermi (1901–1954), the legendary Italian American physicist, gave a colloquium at Columbia University, which was a big attraction to all physicists in New York City. Yalow wanted to attend the colloquium so much that she competed desperately for a seat, and she ended up hanging from the rafters in the top row of the lecture hall, listening as Fermi explained that an atom could split and release energy. It was exciting news that nuclear fission could produce isotopes that could eventually be used in medical research. Yalow was so deeply impressed that she pursued a career later in the application of radioisotopes in medicine.

At Hunter College, Yalow was very unhappy with women professors because they were against combining science and marriage. She said, "Neither of the two women professors I had with the physics department at Hunter did anything to get me along in physics…. In my career, I got help from men, not women."

Yalow wanted to get into medical school, but she knew that she wouldn't be accepted. She said, "American medical schools would not admit Jewish men, let alone women." Instead of choosing medicine, she chose physics. As for discrimination, she said, "Personally, I have not been terribly bothered by it. I have understood that it exists, and it's just one other thing that you have to take into account in what you're doing.... If I wasn't going to do it one way, I'd manage to do it another way."

During her senior year at Hunter College, thanks to the help of Dr. Jerrold Zacharias (1905–1986), physics professor at Hunter College, she obtained a part-time secretarial job with Dr. Rudolf Schoenheimer (1898–1941), a well known biochemist at the College of Physicians and Surgeons of Columbia University. She took this job because she knew that in that capacity she could take some science courses at Columbia. Rosalyn graduated from Hunter College with high honors in physics and chemistry in January of 1941. She then entered a secretarial school to learn stenography. At the same time, she applied for graduate school in physics. Excitingly, she got an offer of a teaching assistantship in physics from the University of Illinois, Champaign-Urbana, the most prestigious school to which she had applied. "It was an achievement beyond belief," she said. She tore up her stenography books, stayed as a secretary until June, and took advantage of enrolling in free physics courses at New York University that summer under governmental auspices. In the fall of 1941 she headed to Illinois.

At the University of Illinois, she was the only woman among the 400 members of the faculty (including teaching assistants) of the College of Engineering. There had not been a woman on the faculty since 1917. One reason she was able to enter the graduate school there was the drafting of young men into the armed forces prior to the United States' involvement in World War II. On the first day of graduate school, she met Aaron Yalow, also a beginning graduate student in physics. The two would eventually marry.

In graduate school, Rosalyn was a half-time assistant teaching freshman physics. Rosalyn experienced subtle gender discrimination, as she recalled. Because as a woman, she was not considered qualified to teach engineers, she could only teach less advanced pre-med students. This was not changed until later when male faculty members were in shortage because of the war.

On December 7, 1941, the Pearl Harbor attack by the Japanese brought the United States into war with Japan. The physics department was decimated by loss of senior faculty to war-related scientific work elsewhere. The campus was filled with young Army and Navy students sent there by their respective services for training. Rosalyn was overloaded with graduate courses, teaching responsibilities, and her experimental thesis that required long hours in the laboratory. She worked hard and managed to obtain her M.S. in 1942 and her Ph.D. degree in nuclear physics in 1945. Her Ph.D. dissertation was *Doubly Ionized K-shell Following Radioactive Decay*. Her major professor was Dr. Maurice Goldharber (b. 1911) who later became director of Brookhaven National Laboratories. Rosalyn was grateful to her major professor and his wife, Gertrude Goldharber (1911–1998), who was also a physicist but had no university position because of Illinois' rule against spouses teaching in the same department.

As mentioned, Rosalyn met Aaron the first day of class. They quickly fell in love. But they could not get married because of the university's rule since both were teaching assistants and technically faculty members. The marriage took place June 6, 1943, when Aaron got a fellowship and was no longer considered a faculty member. When Rosalyn finished her Ph.D. degree, she returned immediately to New York alone to work as assistant engineer, the only woman engineer at the time at the Federal Telecommunications Laboratory, a research laboratory for International Telephone and Telegraph Corporation (ITT). Aaron's thesis was delayed, and later he joined her in the fall of 1945 after he also had obtained his Ph.D. degree. Aaron later became a physics professor at Cooper Union. They first lived in an apartment in Manhattan and later in a small house in the Bronx.

A year later, Rosalyn quit the job at ITT and went back to Hunter College to teach physics to veterans enrolled in a pre-engineering course. She had always been interested in medical research. In the beginning, she volunteered to work for Dr. Edith Quimby (1891–1982), a leading medical physicist at the College of Physicians and Surgeons of Columbia University, to gain experience in the medical applications of radioisotopes. Through her help, she found a part-time job as a consultant in the new Radioisotope Section of the Bronx VA Hospital in 1947. By then radioisotopes were readily available. Rosalyn started to do research with Dr. R. Bernard Roswit. She quickly turned a janitor's closet into one of the first radioisotope laboratories in the United States and generated about eight publications in different areas of clinical investigations. Rosalyn was so interested in the subject that she started working full-time at the VA Hospital in 1950, when Solomon Berson, a medical doctor who completed his residency at the VA Hospital, was appointed to work in the Radioisotopes Unit. They began a wonderful partnership that lasted 22 years.

Initially, radioiodine was used in the study of thyroid physiology and the diagnosis of thyroid disease. The radioisotopically labeled substances were injected into the blood and samples were taken after the injected material had been mixed homogeneously. Yalow and Berson then determined the relative amount of red blood cells and examined them to see whether the anemia was due to an absolute decrease of the number of red blood cells or to an increase in plasma volume caused by cirrhosis or heart failure. They also developed experimental methods to measure the rate of removal of serum protein from the bloodstream and determined the rates of synthesis and degradation of serum protein.

Drs. Yalow and Berson became a remarkable research team. They respected each other and learned from each other. Rosalyn said, "He wanted to be a physicist, and I wanted to be a medical doctor." With a rich knowledge of clinical medicine and experiences, Dr. Berson wanted to improve medical research. And Rosalyn was a superb physicist, chemist, and mathematician. In combination, they became brilliant team investigators with high innovative and critical research capabilities. The collaboration between Yalow and Berson was so successful that they felt that they were on a mission to understand how radioisotopes could be used in human medicine. They never thought of a receiving a Nobel Prize in the beginning, but much fascinating progress kept them excited, and both of them became aware that a big prize would be coming in time.

One of the outstanding studies they jointly conducted was the research on the distribution and degradation of insulin — a small peptide hormone discovered in Canada in 1922 by Frederick Grant Banting (1891–1941), Charles H. Best (1899–1978), and John James R. MacLeod (1876–1935). They administered radioactive-labeled insulin intravenously to diabetics and non-diabetics. They surprisingly found that the diabetics had a slow disappearing rate of insulin because insulin was bound to antibodies in the blood. Because insulin served as an antigen, they developed a new and highly sensitive method to quantitatively determine the concentration of insulin-bound antibodies in the circulation. Reciprocally, they used the same method to measure the concentration of antigen (i.e., insulin) in the blood. This is the basic principle of radioimmunoassay (RIA).

Yalow was extremely good with the required mathematical calculations involved in RIA. This technique is so sensitive that a Swedish scientist commented, "It is like detecting the presence of half a lump of sugar in a lake about 62 miles wide and long and 30 feet deep." In precise terms, RIA can detect a billionth of a gram. There are many advantages of the procedure: all analyses can be done in test tubes, it is not necessary to inject radioactive substances into the body, and only a tiny amount of sample (such as a tenth of a ml of blood) is sufficient for the test. Furthermore, RIA works for virtually every hormone and for a variety of biological important substances. Measurements can be carried in any laboratory with radioactivity counting equipment.

Like any new scientific adventure, in the beginning RIA was faced with resistance. Yalow and Berson published their idea for RIA in 1956 and then spent years developing the concept into a practical test. When Berson gave a speech at the University of Illinois, 29 out of 30 people in the audience thought that he was crazy. There was only one person who appreciated the approach. When Yalow and Berson submitted their first paper to be published in 1959, it was rejected by *Science* and by *The Journal of Clinical Investigation*, because the editors of those journals would not believe that insulin would induce antibodies. Eventually, the paper was published when the word "insulin antibody" was deleted from the title.

Over time, Yalow and Berson published many research papers describing RIA in detail. From time to time, Yalow and Berson also trained a limited number of postdoctoral fellows in their laboratory. They advised many investigators on the RIA technique, which was to be used in laboratories throughout the world.

RIA revolutionized the study of diabetics. By using RIA, medical doctors could separate diabetics into two groups: those who lose the ability to synthesize insulin during childhood, and those who produce plenty of insulin but lose the ability to use it during adulthood. Those two groups of patients should be treated differently. RIA is also used in the study of human growth hormones. These are essential for bone development and growth, but little was known about them before RIA became available. Not limiting themselves to insulin and human growth hormones, Yalow and Berson studied many other hormones including parathyroid hormone, adenocorticotropic hormone (ACTH), and many other substances such as hepatitis B-antigen, enzymes, vitamins, viruses, and drugs within the human body. Eventually, more than one hundred biological substances were measured using RIA.

RIA is used to diagnose conditions caused by hormonal excesses or deficiencies. Yalow and Berson identified people with all kinds of diseases including peptic ulcers, kidney stones, hypertension, hormone-secreting cancers, and other endocrine-related disorders. Berson and Yalow also developed a theory about the biosynthesis of ACTH using RIA. Because of their work, endocrinology became one of the hottest areas of medical research.

RIA contributed greatly to clinical medicine, making advances in the diagnosis and treatment of many human diseases. RIA actually initiated a new science: neuroendocrinology, which is the study of the chemical messengers used by the brain to control the human hormone systems. RIA can pinpoint the concentration of drugs in blood, which is essential in chemotherapy. Drugs need to reach a certain concentration in a patient's blood in order to be effective. If too much of a drug is given, it is toxic, and if not enough is administered, it is ineffective.

In 1968 Berson was appointed professor at the Mount Sinai School of Medicine of the City University of New York, where he was in charge of internal medicine. By then Berson believed that the discovery of RIA was essentially complete, and he wanted to teach medicine, philosophy, and mathematics. This was a disappointment to Yalow. Nevertheless, research collaborations continued, as Berson went to the VA laboratory as much as he could. In 1970 Yalow was made chief of the Nuclear Medicine Service at the VA hospital. In March of 1972 Berson had a slight stroke, and he asked an associate, Eugene Straus, to work with Yalow. Unfortunately, Berson died of a heart attack in April of 1972.

Berson's death was a big blow to Yalow, and she was devastated for more than a year. Yalow then became more determined and worked even harder. Instead of 80 hours a week, she worked 100 hours. She renamed her laboratory the Solomon A. Berson Research Laboratory and continued publishing papers that carried Berson's name. With the new partner, Eugene Straus, 60 articles were published between 1972 and 1976. One of the unique discoveries from Yalow and Straus in that period was that cholecystokinen, a hormone that helps digest fats in the small intestine, is also a synaptic transmitter in the brain, communicating information from one neuron to another. She continued to work at the VA hospital until 1991, when she decided to retire.

In 1975 Yalow was elected to the National Academy of Sciences. The next year, she was the first woman to win the Albert Lasker Award for basic medical research. In 1977 Yalow received a Nobel Prize. Between 1974 and 1977, Yalow received five honorary doctorates. She was elected to membership of the American Academy of Arts and Sciences in 1978. Yalow received more than 50 honorary degrees from American universities and colleges and from universities in Argentina, Canada, Belgium, and France.

In 1968 she was affiliated with the Mt. Sinai School of Medicine as a research professor, and in 1974 her title was changed to that of distinguished research professor. In 1980 she was a distinguished professor at large at the Albert Einstein College of Medicine in Yeshiva University, New York. In 1981 she was an acting chairperson of the Department of Clinical Sciences, Montefiore Medical Center in the Bronx. In 1986 Mt. Sinai named her Solomon A. Berson Distinguished Professor at Large.

Dr. Yalow served as an advisor to important medical committees and as a member of the editorial boards of important journals. She received numerous awards. She was a recipient of the Eli Lilly Award (1961); Gairdner Foundation International Award (1971); Koch Award of the Endocrine Society (1972); A. Cressy Morrison Award in Natural Sciences of the New York Academy of Sciences (1975); Banting Medal of the American Diabetes Association (1978); Scientific Achievement Award of the American Medical Association; American College of Physicians Award for distinguished contributions in science as related to medicine; first William S. Middleton Medical Research Award of the Veterans Administration; Georg Charles de Henest Nuclear

Medicine Pioneer Award in 1986; and in 1988 the National Medal of Science, the nation's highest science award.

Yalow was an extremely hard worker. She came to her laboratory early in the morning and worked until late at night. She would work in the laboratory even when she was sick.

Neither Yalow nor Berson was money-minded. Together they decided not to patent their discovery, which was contradictory to many commercial laboratories that performed RIA. She said, "In my day, scientists didn't patent things. You did it for the people."

When she was asked what she planned to do with the Nobel Prize money, she said that between her husband, children, and laboratory, she had all that she wanted. Her work, she declared, gave her continuous energy.

The marriage between Aaron and Rosalyn was a successful one. Rosalyn commented that Aaron's support was invaluable to her work. Aaron said, "I've served as an extra pair of hands and eyes and another brain." But not, apparently, as an extra cook; Rosalyn did all the cooking. When she traveled, she cooked his meals ahead of time for him to warm. She even kept a Kosher kitchen for him. Neither she nor her parents had kept such a tradition.

During Yalow's high-flying time of research, she bore and raised two children. Her son, Benjamin, was born in 1952, and her daughter, Elanna, was born in 1954. When Benjamin was born, she took seven days off for his birth and nursed Benjamin for ten weeks. She then trained him to sleep during the day and play during the night while she was home. Nine days after the birth of her daughter Elanna, Yalow gave a lecture in Washington, D.C. Despite her busy work schedule, she was an attentive mother. She insisted on being able to have lunch with her children. She moved into a house that was less than a mile from the VA hospital and never moved to a more elegant suburb, which might have made that lunch impossible. She had a sleep-in housekeeper until Benjamin was nine years old. When Elanna entered elementary school, Yalow switched to part-time help but still found time to volunteer for class trips. On the weekend, she took her children to her office to play with equipment and the rabbits, mice, and guinea pigs.

Yalow kept pushing the role of women in science. In her banquet speech after receiving the Nobel, she observed that women were not proportionally represented among the scientists, scholars, and leaders of the world. She thought that women had not achieved to an extent consistent with their abilities mainly because of professional and social discrimination. In her speech she said:

> We cannot expect in the immediate future that all women who seek it will achieve full equality of opportunity. But if women are to start moving

towards that goal, we must believe in ourselves or no one else will believe in us; we must match our aspirations with the competence, courage and determination to succeed; and we must feel a personal responsibility to ease the path for those who came afterwards.

Although Yalow strongly believed in equal opportunity and equal access, she opposed women-only awards and affirmative action programs for women. She turned down the Federal Women's Award in 1961 and the *Ladies' Home Journal* Woman of the Year Prize in 1978. In the presidential address of the Endocrine Society in 1978, she called herself a "non–Establishmentarian." She said that she felt secure enough to be "one of the few chairpersons who dare to be a chairman." She explained that she approached everything aggressively. However, she did express the true meaning of equal opportunity and equal access between men and women. She did advocate paying more attention to child care. She said, "It's a tragedy for society when talented women do not have children.... It is difficult in a field that changes as rapidly as science to drop out for a number of years and then hope to return without major retraining.... When I go out to universities I ask, 'What have you done in the way of day-care centers?'"

*   *   *

Dr. Yalow's career was influenced by the work of Drs. Henri Becquerel (1852–1908) and George Hevesy (1885–1966). Dr. Becquerel was one of the discoverers of radioactivity, and Dr. Hevesy showed how radioisotopes could be used as tracers in chemical and physiological processes. They were scientific progenitors of her career. Another important person who influenced Yalow was Madame Marie Sklodowska Curie (1867–1934). The autobiography of Madame Marie Curie was published by her daughter Ève Curie Labouisse (1904–2007) in 1937. Madame Curie's story had a special meaning for Yalow. She said, "For me, the most important part of the book was that in spite of early rejection, she succeeded. It was in common with my background with my being aggressive." She hosted a five-part dramatic series on the life of Madame Curie, which was aired by the Public Broadcasting Service in 1978.

Dr. Yalow is a very interesting person as characterized by her high energy and uplifting spirit. An extraordinarily sharp intellectual, she was also a devoted wife and mother, as well as a great colleague. When she was asked about the death of Solomon Berson, she expressed sadness that he had not lived to share the Nobel with her. She called her associates and the young research scientists "my professional children." Yalow told her postdocs that she was their professional mother, and Solomon their professional father, and other fellows their brothers and sisters. "We were a protected species," Seymour Glick, once her postdoc, said. She nurtured many potential great scientists. For example, Mildred Spiewak Dresselhaus (1930–) was her first student in 1950. Because of Yalow, Dresselhaus switched her major from elementary education to physics, and then went on to become an MIT professor and a member of the National Academy of Engineering and the National Academy of Sciences. Both Rosalyn and Aaron made it a point to attend seminars or talks given by Dr. Dresselhaus. Dresselhaus said, "Yalow mothered her students, turning them into protégés.... She was like a parent focusing on her child."

Yalow never ignored the importance of family. She often combined family and sciences. She not only took her family to Stockholm for the Nobel festivities, but she also took three Bronx students with her — one from her junior high school, one from Walton High, and one from Hunter College — to write their impressions for their school newspapers.

Yalow could be aggressive, as she admitted herself. She was unpopular among many colleagues in her own field and among scientists on other subjects who had worked with her on professional projects. She was outspoken and held strongly to her opinions. She would fiercely criticize her competitors' works. Even though she nurtured her protégés profoundly, her scathing reviews of her competitors' grant applications and journal articles were devastating. It seems a shame that a scientist of such competence and confidence sometimes made use of such aggressive tactics. Still, she made great contributions in science, had a rich and satisfying personal life, and spoke eloquently for women's equal rights and equal access to opportunities.

Further Reading

Katterman, L. 1999. Rosalyn Sussman Yalow. In *Notable Woman Scientists*. Edited by Pamela Proffitt. Detroit: Gale Group.

McGrayne, S. B. 1993. *Nobel Prize Women in Science: Their Lives, Struggles and Momentous Discoveries*. 2nd ed. Washington DC: Joseph Henry. 333–354.

Odelberg, Wilhelm, ed. 1978. *Les Prix Nobel* (The Nobel Prizes). Stockholm: Nobel Foundation.

Opfell, O. 1978. *The Lady Laureates: Women Who Have Won the Nobel Prize*. Metuchen NJ: Scarecrow. 254–264.

Yalow, Rosalyn. 1977. Nobel Banquet Speech. Dec. 10. http://nobelprize.org/nobel_prizes/medicine/laureates/1977/yalow-speech.html

24

JEWEL PLUMMER COBB
(1924–)

Renowned Cancer Researcher and University Administrator

I know that I was at a constant disadvantage because I was both black and a woman, but I used that as a drive to work hard and succeed. This was the world we lived in; who knows where I would have gone if I had been a white woman?—Jewel Plummer Cobb (1924–)

Jewel Plummer Cobb was a successful teacher, cancer researcher, and administrator. She did valuable work studying the growth of cancer cells and evaluating treatment to fight against cancer. She was a good teacher of biology. She was also a great administrator, running a big university and bringing education to a higher level. She has also contributed to the education of minority students. Her success story proves that hard dedication to one's profession results in success.

Jewel Isadora Plummer was born January 17, 1924, in Chicago, Illinois. Her father was Frank V. Plummer, a physician; her mother was Carribel Cole Plummer, a physical education teacher. Frank Plummer was the first African American to receive the degree of Doctor of Medicine from Cornell University and was elected president of the National Medical Association. He specialized in dermatology, to the degree that black doctors could in the 1920s. He was on the staff at Provident Hospital, which was affiliated with the University of Chicago and had been established just before the turn of the 20th century. He also helped found the Alpha Phi Alpha Fraternity at Cornell. Frank's father was a freed slave and eventually graduated from Howard University in 1898 and became a pharmacist. Carribel studied interpretive dancing and taught dance and physical education in Chicago's schools. She eventually earned a B.A. degree. Both Frank and Carribel cared about Jewel's education and especially encouraged Jewel's interest in science when Jewel was young.

The Plummer family lived in an apartment building and had friends such as Carter G. Woodson (1875–1950), a historian; Arna Bontemps (1902–1973), a writer; Allison Davis (1902–1983), a famous black anthropologist; and Alpha White, the director of the YWCA. There were many other important black American artists and professionals who lived in the vicinity, although the neighborhood was predominantly white. In Dr. Cobb's recollections, she always heard discussions of racial matters in her home. One of the predominant topics of conversation was the lack of recognition of the accomplishments of African Americans. An example was Daniel Hale Williams (1856–1931), who had performed the first open-heart surgery in 1893. Jewel Plummer, therefore, became familiar with the aspirations, successes, and talents of African Americans even at her young age. She also had the advantage of her father's home library, which contained a considerable collection of books and materials about African Americans, scientific journals and magazines, and periodicals of current events. She seemed to be seeded with an ambition that she would produce great accomplishments in her life.

Jewel Plummer attended the Sexton Elementary School, a predominantly white school. However, in 1929–1930, the Chicago Board of Education gerrymandered the school districts so that fewer black children were eligible to attend Sexton. Jewel was transferred to Betsy Ross Elementary School, which was an overcrowded, old, and dilapidated school.

In 1941 Jewel graduated from a public high school in Chicago and enrolled in the University of Michigan. However, her education was a difficult road because of serious racial segregation at the time. Black students there were put into a different dormitory and were not allowed to eat at popular student restaurants near the campus. After a year at Michigan, Jewel decided to transfer to the historically black Talladega College in Alabama where she graduated with a B.A. in biology in 1944. She pursued her graduate education at New York University and obtained her master's degree in 1947 and Ph.D. in 1950, both in cell physiology. Her Ph.D. dissertation was *Mechanisms of Pigment Formation*.

After earning her Ph.D., Cobb entered the National Cancer Institute on a postdoctoral fellowship (1950–1952) at New York's Harlem Hospital. She worked on the growth of cancer cells and the effects of anticancer chemotherapeutical agents against these cells. She designed new experiments to compare the *in vivo* (in the cancer patients) effects of these chemotherapeutic agents with *in vitro* (cells growing in flasks) effects of the same tissues obtained from the patients. In 1952 she left New York to take a teaching job at the University of Illinois Medical School in Chicago.

In 1954 she returned to New York to work at New York University Tissue Culture Research Laboratory. She entered what she called "an exciting phase of basic research in the cancer chemotherapy program." She continued to work on cancer cell growth and the new chemotherapy drugs that were invented to cure cancer. She worked on the effect of drugs such as actinomycin D and 6-mecaptopurine, synthesized by Gertrude Elion (1918–1999). Those were the frontlines of cancer therapy at that time. She helped establish a baseline of knowledge on the chemotherapy of cancer. She continued this line of research for 22 years and published more than fifty books, articles, and other scholarly reports. She eventually became world renowned.

Dr. Cobb was also interested in teaching. In 1960 she took a professorship to teach biology at Sarah Lawrence College in Bronxville, New York, outside of New York City. She stayed at Sarah Lawrence until 1969 and enjoyed the most intensive teaching phase of her career. In 1969 she accepted the appointment as professor of biology and dean of Connecticut College in New London, where she combined teaching, research, and administration. She found that she liked being an administrator. In 1976 she took the job of dean at Douglass College, the women's college of New Jersey's Rutgers University. She stayed in that job until 1981 when she accepted the highest appointment of her career, president of California State University at Fullerton. She managed 24,000 students and 1,000 faculty members. She established many new programs and made the university one of the best state universities in California. She held this position until 1990, when she retired.

After retirement, she served as president emeritus of California State University Fullerton and as trustee professor at California State University, Los Angeles. She also served on several corporate boards. She was also principal investigator of the ACCESS Center, a program designed to encourage economically disadvantaged middle and high school students to pursue careers in mathematics, science, and engineering.

Despite a busy schedule in administration, Dr. Cobb continued to combine scientific research and college teaching and continued to publish frequently. She was also an influential promoter of programs involving women's and minority students' interest in science.

Dr. Cobb was a member of many academic organizations. She was a member of Sigma Xi society, a fellow of the New York Academy of Sciences, a fellow of the National Cancer Institute (1950–1952), a member of the Education Committee of the Tissue Culture Association (1972–1974), and a member of National Science Foundation and Human Resource Commission (1974). She was also a developer and director of the Fifth Year Post Baccalaureate Pre-Med Program at Connecticut College and a member of the Board of Trustees of the Institute of Education Management.

As an educational leader, Dr. Cobb was awarded more than 21 honorary doctorates by schools such as the Medical College of Pennsylvania, Rutgers University, Tuskegee University, Northeastern University, and Rensselaer Polytechnic Institute. She was elected to membership of the National Academy of Science, Institute of Medicine. In 1993 she was honored with a lifetime achievement award by the Academy for her outstanding contributions for the advancement of women and underrepresented minorities. The Academy has also placed her photograph in its hall of distinguished scientists.

Jewel was the only child of her parents and is the third generation of the Plummer family who had high education. She was quite ambitious at a very young age and focused on her studies in order to pursue her goal. Since she belonged to an African American family, she was concerned about the accomplishments of black Americans in general. Although she grew up in a middle class family, her upbringing did not exempt her from society's racist practices at that time. From her childhood, she experienced racial segregation in Chicago's public schools. While attending the University of Michigan, she was forced to stay in segregated housing for three semesters and witnessed the blatant face of racism. In indignation, she transferred to Talladega College. When she applied for graduate school, New York University denied her entry into the program after realizing her racial background. She appeared at the institution armed with her poise and excellent credentials and succeeded in obtaining her teaching fellowship. All these incidents proved that Dr. Cobb did not allow racial prejudice to derail her. While president of the California State University, Fullerton, she initiated many programs. Among her significant accomplishments were the establishment of the first privately funded gerontology center in Orange County, California, and the creation of the first President's Opportunity Program for students from ethnic groups that were not fully represented on campus. She also lobbied the California Legislature for new student housing on the Fullerton campus.

Jewel married Mr. Roy Cobb in 1952. But the marriage wasn't successful, and they divorced in 1967. They had a son who also became a medical doctor and now is working in New Jersey as a radiologist.

* * *

Dr. Cobb maintained focus to achieve her life goal. As a student, she studied hard to obtain good academic records. As a scientist, she pursued research diligently to achieve recognition internationally. As a teacher, she was devoted and successful. As an administrator, she brought the most needed programs to the campus and was remembered as a competent leader.

She never forgot her background. On one occasion, she compared the situation of women to being in a filter, through which the filtrates pass according to the filter's pore size. Women, she said, must pass through filters with smaller pores than those for men. What a remarkable comparison!

Further Reading

Ambrose, Susan A., Kristin A. Dunkle, Barbara B. Lazarus, Indira Nair, and Deborah A. Harkus. 1997. Jewel Plummer Cobb. In *Journeys of Women in Science and Engineering: No Universal Constants*. Philadelphia: Temple University Press. 68–71.

Warren, W. 1999. Jewell Plumber Cobb. In *Black Women Scientists in the United States*. Bloomington: Indiana University Press. 40–49.

25

ALICE SHIH-HOU HUANG
(1939–)

Eminent Molecular Biologist, Educator, and Leader

I don't believe that major paradigm shifts are the results of serendipity.—
Alice S.-H. Huang (1939–)

Alice Huang is well known for her work on the defective interfering particles of virus. She has also done a lot of research on the replication and regulation of viruses. Her work on vesicular stomatitis virus (VSV) led to the discovery of virion-associated RNA-dependent RNA polymerase, which paved the way to David Baltimore's discovery of RNA-dependent DNA polymerase (reverse transcriptase). She has been very active in promoting science education in general and women's scientific careers in particular. She has been a highly visible role model for female students and junior scientists across the country and the world.

Alice was born on March 22, 1939, in Nanchang, the capital city of the province of Jiangxi, China. She was the youngest of four children of Reverend Quentin K. Y. Huang and Grace Betty Soong. Quentin Huang was the second Chinese bishop ordained by the Anglican Episcopal Ministry in China. Grace Betty Soong was an educated, modern Chinese intellectual. After raising four children, she went to nursing school at the age of forty-five and started a new career of her own.

Alice was influenced by her father, who taught her that she could do anything that she wanted to do. At the age of seven, she decided that she wanted to become a physician who could heal human bodies. This desire was intensified when she later witnessed the suffering caused by illnesses of many of her fellow Chinese. While she was growing up, she was also influenced by two teachers. They were her fifth and sixth grade teacher, Elizabeth W. Jackson, and her high school history teacher, Elizabeth Fry. Both women taught her to be dedicated and also instilled a desire to be helpful to others.

In 1949 when Alice was ten years old, China fell to the Communists. The Huangs sent their children to the United States for a more stable life and greater opportunities. Alice attended an Episcopalian boarding school for girls in Burlington, New Jersey, and later at the National Cathedral School in Washington, D.C. Alice was naturalized as a U.S. citizen in her senior year in high school.

Alice received a scholarship to attend Wellesley College in Massachusetts from 1957 to 1959. She subsequently enrolled in a special program at the Johns Hopkins University School of Medicine and obtained her B.A. degree in human biology in 1961. At that time, she had the chance to get into medical school and become a medical doctor. However, she got ill and depressed when she saw a very elderly, sick man in bed with lots of bedsores. She decided that perhaps to be a doctor was not the right goal for her. She realized that saving bodies and preventing people from dying was only one aspect of medicine; there was so much more to it. She discovered that she would like to be an experimentalist rather than a clinical doctor. She remained at Johns Hopkins and pursued her studies in medicine by going to graduate school. She majored in microbiology under the mentorship of Dr. Robert R. Wagner (1923–). She did research on human herpes simplex virus and vesicular stomatitis virus. Her research has contributed greatly to the understanding of the regulation of RNA synthesis. As a graduate student, she was the first to discover the defective interfering (DI) viral particles. She postulated that these mutants played an important role in viral pathogenesis. Her work stimulated research in many viral systems and led to an important avenue for controlling diseases especially for plants. While still a student, she published seven research papers in major journals. She obtained a master's degree in 1963 and a Ph.D. degree in 1966, both in microbiology, from the Johns Hopkins University.

Dr. Alice Huang spent a year as a visiting assistant professor of the National Taiwan University in Taipei. She also gave lectures at the Academia Sinica located in the same city. In 1967 she did her postdoctoral work with Dr. David Baltimore (1938–) at the Salk Institute for Biological Studies in San Diego, California. Soon Alice and David fell in love and were married in 1968 just when Dr. Baltimore was offered an associate professorship at the Massachusetts Institute of Technology (MIT), Cambridge. Dr. Alice Huang took her research to MIT and continued her postdoctoral work for a year. In 1969 Alice became a research associate at the Department of Biology of MIT. The same year, she received a patent for "Defective Interfering Particles." At MIT, she also received another patent for a laboratory method that allowed researchers to test for bacterial adherence, or the ability of bacteria to stick to a surface.

Dr. Huang's research was centered on how viruses replicate. Using the stomatitis virus as a model, she focused on how the RNA synthesis occurred inside of the host. The central dogma of molecular biology at that time was that RNA is made from DNA (transcription), and RNA was later used as transcript for the synthesis of protein (translation). But Drs. Huang and Baltimore found that the RNA viruses would make RNA from RNA by an enzyme called RNA polymerase. Numerous research papers were published on how RNA replication occurs and how it is regulated. These works led to Dr. Baltimore's later discovery of an enzyme (in a mouse leukemia retrovirus) called reverse transcriptase, which can convert RNA to DNA. Dr. Alice Huang played an inspirational role in this big discovery.

Dr. Baltimore's discovery of reverse transcriptase led him to be awarded the Nobel Prize in 1975 along with Dr. Howard Temin (1934–1991) and Renato Delbecco (1914–), who had independently discovered the same enzyme from a chicken retrovirus.

Dr. Alice Huang's study of viral pathogenesis led to many contributions such as the elucidation of the mechanisms of RNA replication and regulation that allowed her to interpret relationships between defective infections and viral diseases.

In 1971 Dr. Huang was offered an assistant professorship of microbiology and molecular genetics at Harvard Medical School, where she started her independent research career. Life at Harvard University was full of challenges for her but generally smooth and rewarding. She became associate professor in 1973 and full professor in 1979. She also served from 1971 until 1973 as a scientific associate in the Channing Laboratory and Department of Medical Microbiology of the Boston City Hospital and director of Infectious Diseases Laboratory at the Children's Hospital in Boston from 1979 to 1989. She devoted her research to how viral replication was regulated. Using a rabies-like virus as a model, she isolated many mutants that were defective in infection, and demonstrated how mutations would affect the total viral population in the host. Her work involved using rhabdoviruses, such as the stromatitis virus, and paramyxoviruses. She illustrated clearly the defective interfering viral pathogenesis. She was also the first to demonstrate that RNA- and DNA-enveloped viruses phenotypically mix their surface glycoproteins resulting in alteration of antigenicity and host range.

With her scientific contribution being recognized, Alice's talents in services and administrative ability have slowly been revealed. She was elected president of the American Society for Microbiology (ASM), which has membership of over 45,000, for the term of 1988-1989. She was the first Asian-born American to head a national scientific society in the United States. She also actively participated in the services of the American Association for the Advancement of Sciences, the American Society for Biochemistry and Molecular Biology, and other scientific organizations. Other professional societies include the Sigma Xi Research Society, Association of Women in Science, Infectious Diseases Society of America (as a fellow), American Society for Virology, American Academy of Microbiology, Society of Chinese Bioscientists of America, and New York Academy of Sciences. She was also appointed trustee of the University of Massachusetts in 1987.

In 1991 Alice accepted the position as dean of the College of Science of New York University. She held this position until 1997. During this period, she was a trustee of Johns Hopkins University in 1992, and in 1993, she was a member of the council of the Johns Hopkins–Nanjing University Center for Chinese and American Studies. Beginning in 1998, she accepted the position as the Senior Councilor for External Relations and Faculty Associate in Biology at the California Institute of Technology, Pasadena, California.

Despite her deep involvement in administration and services, she remained active in basic research. "Acquiring new scientific information and knowledge gives me a sense of exhilaration," she said to her students. She transmitted her excitement in scientific findings to her students and associates who surrounded her. She continued to publish numerous scientific papers while she served as a dean. She has served on the editorial boards *of Intervirology, Archive of Virology, Journal of Virology, Review of Infectious Diseases, ASM News, Microbial Pathogenesis,* and *Journal of Women's Health.*

As a woman administrator, Dr. Alice Huang saw the importance and necessity of being a good spokesperson for women scientists. Throughout Dr. Huang's career, she has been an excellent educator and has always been supportive of science. While at Harvard, she was known for her willingness to take time to speak with students, providing inspiration in the microbiological sciences. At New York University, she was devoted to the development of science programs, research programs, and the research center. She upgraded facilities and resources for research and science education. She pioneered collaboration between active scientists and educators for New York University and other institutions in a citywide training program for K–12 math and science teachers and worked on the development and implementation of new educational technologies at all grade levels. She has always been concerned with promoting diversity in science education.

She has always been involved in initiating participation among women and other under-represented groups. She helped to promote the advancement of women within the ASM. She was a founding member of the Committee on the Status of Women in Microbiology. She has been an extremely effective leader who opened many doors with a leadership style characterized by diplomacy and keen insight, through which she successfully advocated the promotion of the status of women microbiologists within the ASM.

Not limiting her activities to the ASM, Alice is a member of the Committee on Women in Science and Engineering of the National Research Council–National Academy of Sciences and served on the editorial board of the *Journal of Women's Health*, and is a fellow of the Association for Women in Science. Again, she demonstrated her leadership in promoting the status of women and minority scientists in general.

In addition to her regular position, Dr. Huang has often been invited as a guest lecturer or professional speaker on different occasions. For example, she was a visiting Associate Professor of Virology of Rockefeller University, New York, 1975–1976; Professor of Microbiology in Health Sciences and Technology of the Harvard-MIT Program, Cambridge, Massachusetts, 1979–1991; Welcome Visiting Professor in the Basic Medical Sciences of the University of Mississippi, Oxford, Mississippi, 1980; Carl G. Hartford Visiting Professor in Infectious Diseases of Washington University, St. Louis, Missouri; faculty member of the summer seminar, Japanese Association of Mathematical Sciences, 1989; and Visiting Research Professor of New York University, New York, 1998.

Alice never forgets to do service to her mother country, China. She was elected fellow of the Academia Sinica in Taiwan in 1990, the highest honor of a scholarly achievement of the country, and constantly gave advice and actively participates in the development of many scientific programs, from purely consultation to actively directing specific research projects. She also served as a scientific adviser of Diagnostic Biotech (PTE) Ltd. in Singapore 1988–1990. Since 1996 she has been the director of Gene Sing, Inc., of Singapore.

Numerous honors have been bestowed upon Dr. Huang. She was given academic honors of Wellesley College in 1958; Honorary Master of Arts degree from Harvard University in 1980; Honorary Doctor of Science degree from Wheaton College, Massachusetts, in 1982, Mount Holyoke College, Massachusetts, in 1987, and Medical College of Pennsylvania, Philadelphia, in 1991. Other honors and awards include Foundation Lecturer of ASM 1975–1976, and also 1977–1978, Eli Lilly Award in Microbiology and Immunology in 1977, Alumnae Citation Award of the National Cathedral School, Washington, D.C., in 1978, Sixth Hattie Alexander Memorial Lecturer of Columbia University, New York, in 1981, Lee Kuan Yew Distinguished Visitor of National University of Singapore in 1985, Sophie Jones Lecturer of the University of Michigan, 24th Orton K. Stark Lecturer of Miami University, Ohio, in 1988, San Francisco Chinese Hospital Annual Award in 1989, Sigma Delta Epsilon Honorary Women in Science in 1989, New York American Women in Science Award for Outstanding Women Scientist in 1994, Phi Tau Phi Scholastic Honor Society of America in 1997, Fellow of the Association for Women in Science, Achievement Award of the Chinese-American Faculty Association of Southern California in 1999, Alice C. Evans Award of the ASM in 2001.

Alice is particularly interested in education, in career mentoring, and in policy issues related to science and technology. At Cal Tech, she served the board of the Keek Graduate Institute of Applied Life Sciences, the Pacific Council on International Policy, and the Blue Ribbon Committee of the Los Angeles Music Center.

Asked how she would she like to be remembered, she said, "I don't ever try to really guess how history is going to look on different individuals. I hope that those who are alive will remember me with love."

Alice and David have one daughter. Alice now is in Pasadena to continue her career and also help her husband in managing the California Institute of Technology. In her leisure time, she is an avid reader of mystery novels. She enjoys sailing and snorkeling.

* * *

Alice is a paradigm for modern women — tirelessly working on what she believes and endeavoring to achieve it. She said, "As I get older, I realize that the person who's had the most impact on me professionally and whom I admire tremendously is Polly Bunting (1911–1998) — who advised me, 'Keep your eye on your goals. Don't get sidetracked. Get to your position when you can really do some good. — Remember, that when you get to that position, remember that you are still a woman.'" Dr. Alice Huang has a rewarding family life and engages actively in education. Her charisma impresses all who have been associated with her.

APPENDIX: IMPORTANT PERSONS MENTIONED IN THE TEXT

Anderson, James Skelton (1838–1907). British ship owner. Mayor of Aldeburgh. Husband of Elizabeth Garret Anderson (1836–1917).

Anderson, Louisa Garrett (1873–1943). British medical pioneer and social reformer. Daughter of James Skelton and Elizabeth Garrett Anderson. Author of *Elizabeth Garrett Anderson*.

Arkwright, Joseph Arthur (1864–1944). English bacteriologist and physician. Studied meningococci; studied diphtheria and its effect; described stimulus-response variation of coli-typhoid-dysentery organisms.

Arrhenius, Svante August (1884–1927). Swedish chemist and physicist. Nobel laureate in Chemistry, 1903, for theory of electrolyte dissociation. Numerous contributions to chemistry and physics.

Astbury, William T. (1898–1961). British biophysicist. Founding father of X-ray diffraction studies of biological macromolecules.

Avery, Oswald Theodore (1877–1955). Canadian born physician. Researched pneumonia bacteria, their intercellular enzymes, and new serological types causing lobar pneumonia. Discovered (with Alphonse Raymond Dochez) specific soluble substances responsible for immunological activities of pneumococci. Proved (with Maclyn McCarty and Colin MacLeod) that DNA is genetic material.

Baltimore, David (1938–). American molecular biologist. Nobel laureate in Medicine or Physiology, 1975 (with Howard Temin and Renato Dulbecco). President of Rockefeller University, and president of California Institute of Technology.

Bang, Bernhard Lauritz Frederick (1848–1932). Danish physician. Discovered Bang's bacillus, *Brucella abortus*, which caused infectious abortion in cattle and brucellosis in men.

Banting, Frederick Grant (1891–1941). Canadian physician. Discovered (with Charles H. Best) the hormone insulin under the direction of J. J. R. Macleod, 1922. Nobel laureate in Physiology or Medicine, 1923. Studied cortex of adrenal glands, cancer, and silicosis. Stimulated research in aviation medicine.

Barringer, Emily Dunning (1876–1961). American physician. First woman physician (1905) in New York City Hospital and a well known ambulance surgeon.

Bayne-Jones, Stanhope (1888–1970). American physician. Chairman of the Advisory Editorial Board of the History of Preventive Medicine in the U.S. Army in World War II.

Beadle, George Wells (1903–1989). American geneticist. Nobel laureate in Medicine or Physiology, 1958. Researched genetics of Indian corn and cross-over in fruit flies. Co-discovered one gene–one enzyme concept. Pioneer of biochemical genetics.

Beale, Dorothea (1831–1900). English educator. Leader in promoting higher education of women. Head teacher of Cheltenham Ladies College. Established Kensington Society, as well as London Society for Women's Suffrage. Helped establish St. Hilda's College, Oxford. Author of *Textbook of General History, Work and Play in Girl's Schools*.

Beauchamp, Lilia Marie. American medicinal chemist. Researched synthesis of new drugs for biological testing, antiviral agents, acyclovir nucleosides.

Becquerel, Antoine Henri (1852–1908). French physicist. Nobel laureate in Physics, 1903 (with Marie and Pierre Curie). Researched plane polarization of light, phosphorescence, absorption of light by crystals, terrestrial magnetism; discovered radioactivity in uranium and its salts. Discovered Faraday effect in gases.

Benham, Rhoda William (1894–1957). American mycologist. Researched parasitic fungi affecting humans.

Berens, Randolph Lee (1943–). American protozoologist. Studied intermediate metabolic pathways in pathogenic protozoa to find metabolic differences between those organisms and their mammalian hosts.

Bernal, John Desmond (1901–1971). English crystallographic physicist. Contributed to studies of structures of organics, inorganics, liquids, and carbonaceous meteorites in relation to the origin of life, and to studies of structure of simple and complex substances by methods of X-ray crystallography.

Bernard, Claude (1813–1878). French physiologist. Pioneer of modern physiology. Established physiology as an exact science. Discovered glycogenic function of liver and did many human physiological studies.

Berson, Solomon Aaron (1918–1972). American physician. Researched and wrote numerous papers on blood volume measurement with radioisotopes, kinetics of iodine metabolism and thyroid functions, metabolism of albumin-iodine 131; demonstrated insulin antibodies using isotopic methods; developed radioimmunoassay for insulin and other peptide hormones.

Best, Charles Herbert (1899–1978). American physician and educator. Discovered (with F. G. Banting) insulin in 1921. Investigated choline and liver damage; studied insulin and diabetes. Also studied heparin and thrombosis.

Black, James W. (1924–). British analytical pharmacologist. Nobel laureate in Medicine or Physiology, 1988 (with George H. Hitchings and Gertrude B. Elion). Developed two families of drugs: beta-blockers, used for treatment of coronary heart disease, high blood pressure and heart failure, and anti–ulcer histamine receptor blocking drugs including Tagamet.

Blackwell, Antoinette Louisa Brown (1825–1921): First American woman minister of a recognized denomination (Congregational); pioneer suffragist and women's rights advocate.

Blackwell, Emily (1826–1910): American physician. Founded, with sister Elizabeth Blackwell, the Woman's Medical College of New York and the New York Infirmary for Women and Children. Physician and surgeon at New York Infirmary for Women and Children; dean and professor of obstetrics and diseases of women.

Bontemps, Arna Wendell (1902–1973). American novelist, poet, and educator. Author of *Black Thunder* (1936); *Drums at Dusk* (1939); *The Old South: "A Summer Tragedy" and Other Stores of the Thirties* (1973); *God Sends Sunday* (1931); and other works.

Bordet, Jules Jean Vincent (1870–1961). Belgian bacteriologist and physiologist. Founder of the Pasteur Institute in Brussels, Belgium. Nobel laureate in Medicine or Physiology, 1919. Worked in immunology and serology. Gave first description of bacterial hemolysin; discovered (with Octave Gengou) complement-fixation reaction. Discovered bacillus of whooping cough (*Haemophilus pertussis*) and method of immunization.

Bragg, William Lawrence (1890–1971). Australian physicist. Nobel laureate in Physics, 1915, for his work on X-rays and crystal structures.

Brown, Marie Mattingly Meloney. American journalist. Known as Missy Meloney. Editor of *Delineator*, a woman's magazine.

Brown, Wade Hampton (1878–1942). American pathologist. Researched biology of syphilitic infections. Researched constitutional factors and physical environment in relation to heredity and disease.

Bruce, David (1855–1931). Australian physician and bacteriologist. Discovered *Brucella melitensis* causing Malta fever and traced it to milk of Maltese goats. Discovered the cause of sleeping sickness and studied its transmission by tsetse fly. Discovered the cause of nagana (disease of horse and cattle in Central Africa). Investigated Mediterranean fever.

Buckel, C. Annette (1833–1912). American physician. Served as a nurse in the Civil War. Practiced medicine in California.

Bunting-Smith, Mary Ingraham ("Polly") (1911–1998). American microbiologist and educator. President of Radcliffe College (1960–1972).

Burnet, Gilbert (1643–1715). Scottish theologian and historian. Bishop of Salisbury.

Buss, Francis Mary (1827–1894). English educator and reformer. Helped in formation of the Association of Head Mistresses in 1874 and the creation of the Cambridge Training College in 1885 (later the University Department of Education, Hughes Hall). Promoted employment for women.

Butler, Josephine (1828–1906). British women's leader. Advocated women's right to education and many other issues. Opposed the Contagious Diseases Act, which had been introduced in the 1860s in an attempt to reduce venereal disease in the armed forces. Butler objected in principle to laws that applied only to women. Under the terms of these acts, the police could arrest women they believed were prostitutes and could then insist that they have a medical examination. Josephine Butler had considerable sympathy for the plight of prostitutes, who she believed had been forced into the work by low earnings and unemployment. Butler toured the country making speeches criticizing the Contagious Diseases Acts. An outstanding orator, she attracted large audiences. Many people were shocked by the idea of a woman speaking in public about sexual matters.

[Lord] Byron (George Gordon Byron, 6th Lord Byron) (1788–1824): English poet.

Calmette, Albert Leon Charles (1863–1933). French physician and bacteriologist. Discovered (with Alexandre Yersin and Amédée Borrel) serum for snakebite, suc-

cessfully inoculated animals with anti-plague serum. Introduced Calmette's reaction (tuberculin conjunctival test); developed vaccine Bacille-Calmette-Guerin (BCG) for protection from tuberculosis.

Calne, Roy (1930–). British surgeon. Pioneer of transplantation surgery.

Carr, Emma Perry (1880–1972). American physical organic chemist. First recipient of the Garvan Medal (1936). Studied the ultraviolet spectra of organic molecules as a means of investigating their electronic structures.

Cheney, Ednah Dow (1824–1904). American suffragist, civil rights activist, and editor. Author of *Louisa Alcott: Her Life, Letters, and Journal* (1832–1888).

Churchill, Winston Leonard Spencer (1874–1965). British prime minister during World War II. Nobel laureate in Literature, 1953.

Clark, William Mansfield (1884–1964). American chemist. Author of *The Determination of Hydrogen Ions*, 1920; *Topics in Physical Chemistry*, 1948; *Oxidation-Reduction Potentials of Organic System*, 1960. Investigated physical methods in control of pH in oxidation-reduction. Contributed to study of life processes.

Cohn, Mildred (b. 1913). American biochemist and biophysicist. Contributed to the scientific understanding of mechanisms of enzymatic reactions and a method of studying them.

Cole, Rebecca (1846–1922). First African American female medical doctor. Resident physician at the New York Infirmary for Women and Children. Practiced medicine in Columbia, South Carolina. Established Women's Directory Center in Philadelphia.

Cole, Rufus (1872–1966). American physician. Studied infectious diseases and immunity.

Combe, George (1788–1858). British phrenologist. Author of *The Constitution of Man*.

Comstock, John Henry (1849–1931). American entomologist. Researched coccidae and provided basis for determining systematic relationship of these insects. Also provided basis for subsequent systematic work on coccidae in U.S. Studied wing venation of insects, relationship and descent of lepidoptera. Author of *Insect Life: Notes on Entomology; Introduction to Entomology;* and *How to Know the Butterflies.*

Corey, Robert Brainard (1897–1971). American biophysicist. Pioneered work with Linus Pauling on the studies of molecular models of amino acids, proteins and other macromolecules.

Cori, Carl Ferdinand (1896–1984). Austro-Hungarian born American biochemist. Husband of Gerty Cori. Nobel laureate in Medicine or Physiology, 1947 (with G. T. Cori and B. A. Houssay). Contributed to the discovery of glycolysis in liver tumors, isolation of glucose-1-phosphate, and glycogen conversion by phosphorylase. Pioneer in the study of phosphorylation in muscle; the influence of ovariotomy on carbohydrate metabolism in malignant tumors; intestinal absorption; the action of epinephrin on metabolism; and the mechanism of action of insulin.

Crick, Francis H. C. (1916–2004). British biologist. Nobel laureate in Medicine or Physiology, 1962 (with J. D. Watson and M. H. F. Wilkins) in 1962; proposed model for double-helix structure of DNA.

Curie, Pierre (1859–1906). French physicist. Nobel laureate in Physics, 1903 (with Antoine Henri Becquerel and Marie Curie). He also (with his brother Jacques Pierre) discovered piezoelectricity, the electricity generated by squeezing certain crystals, like quartz. Such crystals are used in microphones, broadcasting electronics, stereo systems, and wristwatches.

Dalldorf, Gilbert (b. 1900). American pathologist and virologist. Researched viral disease, poliomyelitis and choriomeningitis; isolated Coxsackie virus from stools of children.

Davies, Emily (1830–1921). British woman activist. Contributed to women's education. Co-founder of Girton College, Cambridge. Helped establish Kensington Society, as well as London Society for Women's Suffrage. Author of *Higher Education of Women* (1866); *Thought on Some Questions Relating to Women* (1910).

Davis, Allison (1902–1983). American anthropologist. Author of *Leadership, Love and Aggression* (1983); *Rebellion or Revolution* (1968); *The Crisis of the Negro Intellectual* (1967); *The Psychology of the Child in the Middle Class* (1968); *Deep-South: A Social Anthropological Study of Caste and Class* (1941); and other works.

Dawson, Martin Henry (1896–1945). American physician. First American in the developmental study of penicillin. Dean of Yale University School of Medicine, 1935–1940. Jordan, Edwin Oakes (1866–1936). American bacteriologist. Author of *General Bacteriology,* 1908; *Food Poisoning,* 1917, 2nd edition 1931; *A Pioneer of Public Health — W. T. Sedgwick* (with G. C. Whipple and C. E. A. Winslow), 1924; *Epidemic Influenza* (with I. S. Falk), 1927; *The Newer Knowledge of Bacteriology and Immunology,* 1928. Researched bacteriology, food poisoning, typhoid fever, influenza, and self-purification of streams.

Debierne, André (1874–1949). French physicist and chemist. Discovered radioactive actinium in 1899. André Debierne was reported to be deeply in love with Marie Curie.

De Duve, Christian Rene (1917–). Belgian biochemist and cell biologist. Researched insulin and glucagon. Developed cell fractionation methods and discovered lysosomes and peroxisomes and their functions. Nobel laureate in Physiology or Medicine, 1974 (with Albert Claude and George Palade).

Delamater, John J. (1787–1867). American physician. Chair of Materia Medica and Pharmacy in the Berkshire Medical Institution at Pittsfield, Massachusetts (1823). First surgeon in America to perform excision of the scapula. Taught many medical subjects in many different medical schools.

Dickens, Charles (1812–1870). English novelist.

Dochez, Alphonse Raymond (1882–1964). American physician. Researched pneumonia and the common cold, prepared specific anticariatinal serum.

Doisy, Edward (1893–1986). American biochemist. Did research on vitamin K and insulin; contributed to the knowledge of antibiotics, blood buffer system, and bile acid metabolism. Author (with Edgar Allen and C. H. Danforth) of *Sex and Internal Secretions*. Nobel laureate in Medicine or Physiology, 1943 (with Henrik Dam).

Dolley, Sarah Reed Adamson (1929–1909). American physician. Co-founder of one of the first general women's medical societies in the United States, the Practitioners Society of Rochester, New York.

Dopter, Charles (b. 1873). French physician. Worked at Pasteur Institute 1908–1939.

Dresselhaus, Mildred Spiewak (1930–). American physicist and engineer. Researched various areas of solid-state physics and application; electronic structure and properties of graphite and its intercalation compounds; carbon fibers and other novel forms of carbon, such as fullerenes and carbon nanotubes; porous carbon materials; and low dimensional thermoelectricity.

Duclaux, Emile (1840–1904). French biochemist, bacteriologist. Collaborator and successor of Louis Pasteur. Researched and published on diseases of plants and microbes; compared surface tension with stretched elastic membrane; studied flow in capillaries.

Dulbecco, Renato (1914–). American molecular biologist. Nobel laureate in Medicine or Physiology, 1975 (with David Baltimore and Howard Temin).

Ehrlich, Paul (1854–1915). German physician. Proposed a theory of immunity in which antibodies are responsible for immunity (1890); formulated side chain theory of antibody formation (1897); synthesized a magic bullet for syphilis (1912). Nobel laureate in Medicine or Physiology, 1908 (with Elie Metchnikoff).

Einstein, Albert (1879–1955). Theoretical physicist. Nobel laureate in Physics, 1921. Numerous contributions to physics, well known for theory of relativity.

Epictetus (c.55–c.135). Greek philosopher. Exponent of Stoicism.

Falco, Elvira Allegra (b. 1918). American experimental clinical chemist. Researched the chemistry of purine and pyrimidine antagonists, and the synthesis of anti-malarial Daraprin, antibacterial Trimethoprim, and uricosuric agent Allopurinol.

Falk, Isidore Sydney (1899–1984). American health economist. Studied and published statistics in diseases, costs, improvement of medical care; national health and social security legislation.

Farr, William (1807–1883). English physician and statistician. Laid foundation for vital statistics in England.

Fawcett, Henry (1833–1884). British economist and politician. Author of *Manual of Political Economy* (1863). Achieved several important improvements in the postal system.

Fawcett, Millicent (1847–1929). British writer and woman activist. Leader of National Union of Women's Suffrage Societies. Helped establish Newnham College in Cambridge. Author of *Political Economy for Beginners*; *Essays and Lectures on Political Subjects*; *The Women's Victory and After*; *What I Remember*; and *Josephine Butler*.

Fermi, Enrico (1901–1954). Italian physicist. Nobel laureate in Physics, 1938. Investigated formation of artificial radioactive substances; first to bring about nuclear transformations of heavy elements by neutron bombardment; developed statistical model of atom; named neutrino that Wolfgang Pauli postulated. Responsible for construction of first atomic pile (nuclear reactors). Helped develop atomic bomb. Worked on high energy physics including pion-nucleon interactions; developed theory of cosmic ray origin; worked on quantum electrodynamics; investigated theory of hyperfine structures of spectrum lines. Fermium, an artificially formed element, is named in his honor.

Fielding, Henry (1707–1754). English playwright and journalist. Wrote a series of farces, novels, operas and light comedies. Best known for his novel *The History of Tom Jones, a Foundling*.

Fleming, Alexander (1881–1955). British microbiologist. Discovered the antimicrobial substance lysozyme in 1921 and penicillin in 1928. Nobel laureate in Medicine or Physiology (with H. W. Florey and Ernst Chain) in 1945.

Flexner, Simon (1863–1946). American

pathologist. Identified the virus that causes poliomyelitis (1909). Other research areas: pathology of toxalbumin and intoxication; biochemistry of snake venoms; experimental pancreatitis and fat necrosis; epidemic encephalitis. Developed Flexner's serum for cerebrospinal meningitis. Discovered dysentery bacillus.

Fowler, Lorenzo Niles (1811–1896). American phrenologist. Author of *Synopsis and Phyrenology and Physiology* (1844); *Marriage, Its History and Philosophy, with Directions for Happy Marriages* (1846); *Lectures on Man.*

Fowler, Orson Squire (1809–1887). American phrenologist. Lectured and wrote on phrenology, preservation of health, public education, and social reforms. Editor, publisher of *America Phrenological Journal.*

Franklin, Benjamin (1706–1790). American statesman, writer, and discoverer. Performed the famous kite experiment to test the properties of electricity. One of those involved in the writing of the Declaration of Independence. First postmaster general of the U.S.

Galilei, Galileo (1564–1642). Italian astronomer, mathematician, and physicist. Considered the founder of modern science. Numerous contributions to physics, mathematics, and astronomy.

Gall, Joseph (1757–1828). Viennese physician. Founder of phrenology.

Garrison, William Lloyd (1805–1879). American abolitionist. Helped found the American Anti-Slavery Society. Founder of the newspaper *The Liberator.*

Gay, John (1685–1732). English poet and dramatist.

George I (1660–1727). King of England (1714–1727).

Goeppert-Mayer, Maria (1906–1972). German physicist. Nobel aureate in Physics (with Hans Jensen and Eugene Wigner) for work on the shell theory of the atomic nucleus.

Goldhaber, Gertrude Scharff (1911–1998). German physicist. Researched identity of beta particles with atomic electrons, ferromagnetism, neutron physics, photoneutrons, neutrons from spontaneous

fission of uranium, nuclear isomers, systematics of nuclear levels; did tests of parity violation in strong interactions.

Goldhaber, Maurice (b. 1911). Austrian physicist. Contributed to numerous articles on neutron physics, radioactivity, nuclear isomers, nuclear photoelectric effects, nuclear models, and fundamental particles.

Greene, Harry Sylvestre Nutting (b. 1904). American pathologist. Researched cancer transplantation.

Gregory, Samuel (1813–1872). American philanthropist. Founded the New England Female Medical College in Boston, first institution in the world for the exclusive medical education of women. Secretary of the college until his death. In 1874 this college was merged with the medical school of Boston University.

Griffith, Frederick (1879–1941). British bacteriologist. Studied the virulence of pneumococci, discovered bacterial transformation.

Guillemin, Roger (1924–). French physiologist. Researched physiology and isolated hypothalamic hormones. Nobel laureate in Medicine or Physiology, 1977 (with R. Yalow and V. Schally).

Hahn, Otto (1879–1968). German physical chemist. Nobel laureate in Chemistry, 1944. Did important work on nuclear fission; discovered protactinium and several trans-uranium elements from atomic number 94 to 96; obtained experimental evidence of nuclear fission in uranium, noting rare gas krypton as product.

Harding, Warren (1865–1903). 29th president of the United States of America (1921–1923).

Hastings, Edwin George (1872–1953). American agricultural bacteriologist and educator. Did research on dairy microbiology and livestock sanitation.

Heinzen, Carl Peter (1809–1880). Radical German-American journalist. Fled to Switzerland in 1844, returned to Germany to take part in the Baden campaign in 1848. Fled to the United States and became publisher of the *Pioneer,* an uncompromising radical newspaper.

Hevesy, George Charles de (1885–1966).

Hungarian physicist. Researched the use of radium and lead isotope. Pioneer work in the use of isotopic indicator in inorganic and life sciences. Studied neutron bombardment of the element, effect of X-ray on the formation of nucleic acid in tumors and in normal organs, iron transport; discovered new element hafnium; author of several important books related to radiochemistry.

Hitchings, George H. (1905–1998). American chemotherapist. Invented therapeutic agents including pyrimethamine for malaria, mercaptopurine for leukemia, diaviridine for coccidiosis, azathioprine for organ transplantations and autoimmune diseases, allopurinol for gout and hyperuricemia; drugs based on rational specific biochemical modifications. Nobel laureate in Medicine or Physiology, 1988 (with James Black and Gertrude Elion).

Hodgkin, Dorothy Crowfoot (1910–1994). British chemist. Nobel laureate in Chemistry, 1964, for her research on the structure of vitamin B_{12} using X-ray crystallographic analysis.

Horace (65–8 B.C.E.). Original name was Quintus Horatius Flaccus. Roman poet.

· Houssay, Bernardo Albert (1887–1971). Argentinean physiologist. Nobel laureate in Medicine or Physiology, 1947 (with Gerty Cori and Carl Cori). Researched endocrinology, physiology, and pharmacology. Investigated relationship of hypophysis gland to carbohydrate metabolism especially with diabetes. Demonstrated that a hormone secreted by the pituitary prevented metabolism of sugar and injection of pituitary extract induced symptoms of diabetes. Studied the physiology of circulation, digestion, and the nervous system. Also studied snake and spider toxins.

James, L. Stanley (1925–1994). New Zealand physician. One of the founders of modern perinatology and a pioneer researcher in the physiology of newborn infants. Recipient of the E. Mead Johnson Award and the Virginia Apgar Award from the American Academy of Pediatrics, and the Ronald McDonald Children's Charity Award.

Jenner, Edward (1749–1823). English physician. Developed cowpox vaccination against smallpox. Pioneer of animal behavior study.

Jex-Blake, Sophia (1840–1912). English physician. Co-founded London School of Medicine for Women with Dr. Elizabeth Anderson. Founded Edinburgh School of Medicine for Women. A women's suffrage supporter.

Joliot-Curie, Irène (1897–1956). Daughter of Pierre and Marie Curie. Discovered that radioactive elements could be prepared from a stable element by bombarding the stable element with alpha particles. Nobel laureate in Chemistry, 1935 (with Frédéric Joliot).

Joliot-Curie, Frédéric (1900–1958). French physicist. Discovered artificial radiation. Nobel laureate in Chemistry, 1935 (with Irène Joliot-Curie).

Kendrew, John Cowdery (1917–1971). British biophysicist. Demonstrated the three-dimensional model of myoglobin. Nobel prize laureate in Chemistry, 1962 (with Max F. Perutz).

Klug, Aaron (1926–). South African chemist. Nobel laureate in Chemistry, 1982.

Krenitsky, Thomas Anthony (1938–). American biochemist. Researched specificities, mechanisms, and phylogenetic relationships of the enzymes including hydroxylating enzymes, ribosyltransferases, phosphoribosyl-transferases, nucleoside and nucleotide kinases, and nucleotide interconverting enzymes.

Ledingham, John C. G. (1875–1944). British bacteriologist. Author (with J. A. Arkwright) of *Carrier Problem in Infectious Diseases*, 1912. Numerous articles on role of carrier in spread of typhoid fever. Proved existence of disease kala-azar in China.

[Lord] Kevin William Thomson (1st Baron Kelvin) (1824–1907). Scottish mathematician and physicist. Did important work in almost every branch of physical sciences.

Kitasato, Shibasaburo (1856–1931). Japanese bacteriologist. Well known for his work on *Clostridium tetani* and tetanus toxin. Developed diphtheria antitoxin (with E. von Behring). Isolated bacilli causing anthrax and dysentery. Worked in social hygiene.

Kluyver, Albert Jan (1888–1956). Pioneer Dutch microbiologist, well known for his research on fermentation and theory of biochemical unity of microorganisms.

Koch, Robert (1843–1910). German microbiologist, physician. Studied anthrax, tuberculosis, cholera in Asia and Africa. Father of medical microbiology. Nobel laureate in Medicine or Physiology, 1905.

Kornberg, Arthur (b. 1918). American biochemist. Nobel laureate in Physiology or Medicine, 1959 (with S. Ochoa). Discovered DNA polymerase. Studied the synthesis of DNA and biosynthesis of NAD and FAD.

Labouisse, Ève Curie (1904–). French writer and musician. Daughter of Marie and Pierre Curie. Author of *Madame Curie* and *Journey Among Warriors.*

Labouisse, Henry R. (1904–1987). American diplomat. Husband of Ève Curie. Director of the United Nations' Children's Fund and received on its behalf the Nobel Peace Price (1965).

Langevin, Paul (1872–1946). French physicist. Studied molecular structure of gases, analyzed secondary emissions of X-ray from metals exposed to radiation. Had a theory of magnetism. Did research on piezoelectricity, piezoceramics, underwater sonar for submarine detection, and other topics.

Lederberg, Joshua (1925–). American geneticist. Pioneer of microbial genetics. Nobel laureate in Medicine or Physiology, 1958.

Leloir, Luis Federico (1906–1987). Argentine biochemist. Nobel laureate in Chemistry, 1970. Discovered sugar nucleotides and their roles in the biosynthesis of carbohydrates.

Levi-Montalcini, Rita (1909–). Italian biochemist. Nobel laureate in Medicine or Physiology, 1986 (with Stanley Cohen), for work on the growth of cells in the peripheral nervous system.

Lincoln, Abraham (1809–1865). 16th president of the United States of America.

Longfellow, Henry Wadsworth (1807–1882). American poet.

Macleod, John James Rickard (1876–1935). Scottish physiologist. With F. G. Banting and Charles H. Best, discovered insulin (1922). Nobel laureate in Medicine or Physiology, 1923 (with F. G. Banting). Numerous research papers on metabolism, physiology of respiration, lactic acid metabolism, chemistry of TB bacillus, and biochemistry of carbohydrates. Author of *Diabetes, Its Physiological Pathology* (1913); *Fundamentals of Physiology* (1916); *Carbohydrate Metabolism and Insulin* (1926); *The Fuel of Life* (1928).

Marr, J. Joseph (1938–). American medicinal molecular biologist. Research on metabolic regulation in microorganisms and its relationship to the pathogenesis of intracellular infections in humans. Author (with Joseph J. Marr, Timothy W. Nelsen and Richard W. Komuniecki) of *Molecular Medical Parasitology*, 2002, and (with Robert F. Boyd) *Medical Microbiology*, 1980.

McClintock, Barbara (1902–1992). American geneticist. Discovered transposons. Nobel laureate in Medicine or Physiology, 1983.

McCollum, Elmer Verner (1879–1967). American physiologist and chemist. Discovered vitamins A and D; developed methods of biological analysis of foodstuff, synthesized several pyrimidines. Author of *Text Book of Organic Chemistry for Medical Students*, 1916; *Newer Knowledge of Nutrition*, 1918, 5th edition, 1939; *The American Home Diet*, 1919; *Food Nutrition and Health*, 1933; *History of Nutrition*, 1957; *From Kansas Farm Boy to Scientist*, 1964.

McCormick, Cyrus Hall (1809–1884). American inventor. Invented and patented hillside plough (1831); patented reaping machine (1834); added mowing attachment to reaper (1950); developed self-raking device, hand binding harvester, wire-binder, twine-binder (1860). Owner *of Chicago Times* (1860); publisher (1860–1861).

McMechan, Francis H. (1879–1939). American anesthesiologist. Established the first anesthesiological journal: *Current Researches in Anesthesia and Analgesia.*

Meitner, Lise (1878–1968). Austrian physicist. Studied nuclear isomerism; found four radioactive elements resulting from neutron bombardment of uranium; predicted chain reactions that contributed to atomic bomb development; split uranium nucleus (with Otto Frisch).

Merrick, Myra King (1825–1899). American physician. First woman physician in Ohio. Helped establish Homeopathic Hospital College for Women in 1887.

Metz, Charles William (1889–1975). American zoologist. Researched cytogenetics with emphasis on nature of chromosomes and their role in heredity, development, sex determination, and evolution.

Meyer, Karl (b. 1899). American biochemist. Researched structure and chemical activities of lysozyme, hyaluronic acid, chondroitin sulfates, and keratosulfates; mechanism of hyaluronidases, patterns of distribution of mucopolysaccharides in connective tissues and their changes with aging.

Mill, John Stuart (1806–1873). British economist and philosopher. Author of *System of Logics,* 1843; *Essays on Some Unsettled Questions in Politics,* 1844; *Principles of Political Economy,* 1848; *Essays on Liberty,* 1859; and other works.

Mitchell, Maria (1818–1889). American astronomer, and educator. Discovered a new comet in 1847. First woman elected to Membership of the American Academy of Arts and Sciences in 1848. First woman professor of astronomy, Vassar College, 1865–1888.

Mittag-Leffler, Magnus Gösta (1846–1927). Swedish mathematician. Founded *Acta Mathematica.* Made important contributions to analysis (including Mittag-Leffler theorem on single-valued functions) and linear differentiation equations.

Morgan, Thomas Hunt (1866–1945). American zoologist. One of the founders of modern genetics. Nobel laureate in Medicine or Physiology, 1933. Author of *Regeneration* (1903), *Experimental Zoology* (1907), *Heredity and Sex* (1913), *Mechanism of Mendelian Heredity (*1915), *Critique of the Theory of Evolution* (1916), *The Physical Basis of Heredity* (1919), *The The-*ory *of Gene* (1926), *Experimental Embryology* (1927), *The Scientific Basis of Evolution* (1932), *Embryology and Genetics* (1933). Numerous publications on biology and embryological subjects. Using Drosophila, demonstrated physical basis of heredity and importance of genes, described phenomena of linkage and crossing over along chromosome, proved linear arrangement of genes along chromosome. Other research and publications on development, experimental embryology, regeneration, evolution, and adaptation.

Mott, James (1788–1868). American abolitionist. Member of the Anti-slavery Society in 1833. Believed in greater rights for women. Founder of Swarthmore College in 1864. Author of *Three Months in Great Britain.*

Mott, Lucretia (1793–1880). American reformer. Spoke on temperance, peace, women's rights, and abolition.

Murray, Joseph Edward (1919–). American surgeon. Nobel laureate of Medicine or Physiology, 1990 (with E. Donnall Thomas).

Newton, Isaac (1642–1727). English mathematician, physicist, and astronomer. Pioneer of modern science. Well known for the discovery of gravity.

Nightingale, Florence (1820–1910). English nurse. Founder of modern nursing education. Pioneered the use of statistical approaches for medical studies and improved health measures.

Norrish, Ronald George Wreyford (1897–1978). English physical chemist. Nobel laureate in Chemistry, 1967 (with M. Eigen and G. Porter). Researched extremely fast chemical reactions by disturbing chemical equilibrium with short energy pulses; made analysis of reactions of one ten billionth of a second possible.

Ochoa, Severo (1905–2000). Biochemist. Nobel laureate in Physiology or Medicine, 1959 (with A. Kornberg). Researched intermediate metabolism, enzymatic reactions of carbohydrates and fatty acid metabolism. First to synthesize nucleic acid in a test tube.

[Lord] Palmerston (Henry John Temple, 3rd

Viscount Palmerston) (1784–1865). English statesman. Served as secretary of war under five prime ministers. Influenced foreign affairs from 1830 to 1865; supported liberal and national causes in Europe.

Papper, Emanuel Martin (1915–2002). American anesthesiologist. Researched and published developmental concepts of general anesthesia; studied metabolism and effects of anesthetics.

Park, William Hallock (1863–1939). American physician and bacteriologist. Author of *Pathogenic Microorganisms*, 10th edition, 1933; *Public Health Hygiene*, 2nd edition, 1927; *Who's Who Among the Microbes*, 1929. Developed a diphtheria antitoxin; improved milk purification; studied child health; organized first municipal health laboratory in New York City. Researched public health effects of tuberculosis, pneumonia, diphtheria, poliomyelitis, etc.

Parker, Theodore (1810–1860).Great American preacher and abolitionist. His teaching had a great influence on the movement of the emancipation of slaves.

Pasteur, Louis (1822–1895). French chemist, microbiologist. Studied yeast fermentation. Studied many diseases including anthrax, pebrine, and rabies. Disproved the fallacy of spontaneous generation.

Pauling, Linus (1901–1994). American chemist. Nobel laureate in Chemistry, 1954, and in Peace, 1963).

Penn, William Fletter. American physician. A brother of Irvine Garland Penn (1867–1930), renowned teacher, editor, and author.

Perey, Marguerite (1909–1975). French physicist. Assistant to Marie Curie. Discovered element 87 and named it francium.

Perrin, Jean (1870–1942). French physicist. Researched Brownian motion of minute particles suspended in liquids, verified Albert Einstein's explanation of the phenomenon and confirmed the atomic nature of matter. Nobel laureate in Physics, 1926.

Perutz, Max (1914–2002). British biochemist. Nobel laureate in Chemistry, 1962 (with John Kendrew). Illustrated the structure of proteins.

Phillips, Wendell (1811–1884). American abolitionist, friend of William Lloyd Garrison and President Abraham Lincoln (1809–1865). Exerted a great influence on the emancipation of slaves during the American Civil War (1861–1865).

Pope, Alexander (1688–1744). English poet, critic, and satirist.

Quetélet, Lambert-Adolphe-Jacques (1796–1874). Belgian statistician and astronomer. Founder of the observatory of Brussels. Author of *Astronomie Elémentaire*, 1826; *Sur l'homme et le dévelopment de ses facultés*, 1835; *Du système social et des lois qui le régissent*, 1845; and *L'Anthropométrie*, 1871. Pioneer in statistics; helped develop uniformity and comparability in international statistics; applied mathematical methods of averages and probabilities to the study of man; developed idea of "average man" as well as that of "vital statistics"; studied meteoric showers; developed methods of simultaneous observations of astronomical meteorological geodetic phenomena at various points through Europe.

Quimby, Edith (1891–1982). American biophysicist. Researched and wrote numerous papers on radiation physics and radiobiology.

Randall, John Turton (1905–1984). English biophysicist. Researched luminescence of solids, structure of collagen, biophysics of cilia; joint discoverer of cavity magnetron.

Rhazes (860–923 or 932). Persian physician, philosopher and religious critic, known as Ibn-Zakariya, also al Razi or Razi. Considered the Islamic Hippocrates. First to use animal gut for sutures, plaster of Paris for casts. Author of *Kitah al-Mansuri and Kitah al-hawi* (meaning *Comprehensive Book*).

Rivers, Thomas M. (1887–1963). American bacteriologist and virologist. Researched measles and pneumonia. Discovered the parainfluenzae bacillus and cultured vaccine virus for human use. Coordinated research on poliomyelitis.

Roller, Duane Emerson (1894–1965). American physicist. Author of *Physical Termi-*

nology; *Mechanics, Molecular Physics, Heat and Sound; Early Development of the Concept of Temperature and Heat; Early History of the Concept of Electric Charge.* Contributed to numerous articles on experimental physics and history, language, and teaching of physics. Editor of *American Journal of Physics,* 1933–1949.

Rosahn, Paul Dolin (1903–). American pathologist. Researched biology of syphilis, biology of cancer, biometrics, hematology, Letters-Siwe's disease, and hyaline membrane diseases.

Rosenblum, Salomon (b. 1889). French physicist. Studied alpha ray. Author of *Origine des rayons, gamma, structure fine du spectre magnétique des rayons alpha/ parm.*

Rutherford, Ernst (1871–1937). New Zealand physicist. Nobel laureate in Chemistry, 1908. Contributed in numerous ways to nuclear physics research.

Sabin, Florence Rena (1871–1953). American anatomist. Discovered origin and process of lymphatic system; developed methods of studying living cells. Author of *An Atlas of the Medulla and Mid-Brain.*

Schaeffer, Howard (1927–). American medicinal chemist. Researched enzyme inhibition, kinetics, stereochemistry, and antiviral chemotherapy. Synthesized acyclovir.

Schally, Andrew V. (1926–). Polish biochemist. Studied ACTH and adrenal cortical steroids' transformation and endocrine activity; hypothalamus hormone; corticotrophin releasing factor; and other topics. Nobel laureate in Medicine or Physiology, 1977 (with Roger Guillemin and Rosalyn Yalow).

Schoenheimer, Rudolf (1898–1941). American biochemist. Introduced isotopic tracers in biochemical research. Used fat molecules that contained deuterium to study fat of animals, found that ingested fat was stored and stored fat was used. Used heavy isotope of nitrogen to study amino acids.

Sedgwick, William Thompson (1855–1921). American biologist. Author of *Principles of Sanitary Science and Public Health* (1902). Coauthor of *General Biology*

(1886), *The Human Mechanism* (1906), and *A Short History of Science* (1917). Early advocate of pasteurization of milk; demonstrated use of chlorine to disinfect water and sewage. Traced typhoid epidemics to polluted brooks and contaminated milk supply.

Semmelweis, Ignatz (1818–1865). Hungarian physician. Proved puerperal fever contagious.

Sewall, Lucy E. (1837–1890). American physician. Student of Dr. Marie Zakrzewska at the New England Female Medical College and a leader of the women's medical movement.

Sewall, Samuel Edmund. Lucy E. Sewall's father, a distinguished Bostonian.

Sloane, Hans (1660–1753). English botanist and physician. Author of *Natural History of Jamaica,* 1707–1723.

Spurzheim, Johann C. (1776–1832). British phrenologist. First coined the term phrenology. Believed that the skull had 37 "powers" corresponding to 37 organs. Author of many phrenology-related writings.

Stanton, Elizabeth Cady (1815–1902). Leader of American women's rights movement.

Stillingfleet, Benjamin (1702–1771). English botanist and writer.

Strassman, Fritz (1902–1980). German physical chemist. Researched nuclear chemistry, nuclear fission, radioisotope of uranium and thorium.

Sutherland, Earl Wilbur, Jr. (1915–1974). American biochemist and pharmacologist. Nobel laureate in Physiology or Medicine, 1971. Discovered cyclic AMP (adenosine 3,'5'-monophosphate) and its role and mechanisms by which many hormones exert control over metabolic processes in the human body.

Swift, Homer Fordyce (1881–1953). American physician. Author of *Forchheimer's Therapeusis of Internal Diseases, Practical Treatment* (Musser and Kelly), *Nelson's Loose-Leaf Medicine, Oxford Loose-Leaf Medicine, Text-Book of Medicine* (Cecil), *Bacterial and Mycotic Infections of Men* (Dubos). Researched treatment of syphilis of central nervous system, rheumatic fever, streptococcal infections, and trench fever.

Tatum, Edward Lawrie (1909–1975). American biochemist and geneticist. Nobel laureate in Medicine or Physiology, 1958 (with George Beadle and Joshua Lederberg). Co-discovered one gene–one enzyme concept. Pioneered studies on genetic mutations in Neurospora.

Temin, Howard (1934–1994). American molecular oncologist. Nobel laureate in Medicine or Physiology, 1975 (with David Baltimore and Renato Dulbecco). Independently discovered reverse transcriptase.

Teresa (1910–1997). Generally called Mother Teresa or Theresa. Original name Agnes Gonxha Bojaxhiu. Great humanitarian. Born in Skopje, Macedonia. In Calcutta, India, founded an order of nuns called the Missionaries of Charity (1950) and the Nirmal Hriday Home for the Dying in a former temple (1952). Nobel laureate in Peace, 1979.

Trall, Russell Thacher (1812–1877). American hydropathist. Founder of American Hygeio-Therapeutic College. Author of many publications such as *Hydropathic Encyclopedia* (1852); *Sexual Physiology* (1866); *Digestion and Dyspepsia* (1874); *Popular Physiology* (1875).

Van Niel, Cornelius Bernardus (1897–1895). American pioneer microbiologist, well known for his research on bacterial photosynthesis, general microbiology, and biochemistry of microorganisms; an influential microbiological educator.

Volhard, Christiane Nusslein (1942–). German biochemist. Studied the genetic makeup of the fruit fly; identified genes responsible for specific biological characteristics in an organism. Nobel laureate in Medicine or Physiology, 1995 (with Edward B. Lewis).

von Behring, Emil (1854–1917). German physician. Developed diphtheria antitoxin (with S. Kitasato). Nobel laureate in Medicine or Physiology, 1901.

Wadsworth, Augustus B. (1872–1954). American physician. First director of the Division of Laboratories and Research of the New York State Department of Health. Researched pneumonia.

Wagner, Robert Roderick (1923–). American virologist. Researched biochemistry of viruses and cell biology of cancer.

Waksman, Selman A. (1888–1973). American soil microbiologist. Pioneered antibiotics research. Involved in the discovery of streptomycin and many other antibiotics. Nobel laureate in Medicine or Physiology, 1952.

Waters, Ralph Miltons (1883–1979). American anesthesiologist. First clinical use (with others) of cyclopropane as anesthesia. Studied anesthetic drugs, anesthetic inhalation equipment, chloroform, nitrous oxide, etc.

Watson, James D. (1928–). American biologist. Nobel laureate in Medicine or Physiology, 1962) (with F. H. C. Crick and M. H. F. Wilkins); proposed model for double-helix structure of DNA.

Welch, William Henry (1850–1934). American pathologist. Discovered *Staphylococcus epidermidis albus* (or called *Micrococcus albus*) and studied its relationship to wound infection. Studied the pathology of diphtheria. Discovered the causative agent of gas gangrene.

Wendell, Stanley M (1904–1971). American biochemist. Nobel laureate in Chemistry, 1946 (with James B. Sumner and John H. Northrop), for work in the purification and crystallization of viruses and the demonstration of their molecular structure.

West, Harold D. (1904–1974). American scientist and educator. Ph.D. University of Illinois, 1937. Researched the synthesis of the essential amino acid threonine, helped discover the antibiotic eucerine. One of the first scientists to use radioisotope to locate infections and tumor. President of Meharry Medical College (1952–1965). Honorary doctorates from Morris Brown College (1955) and Meharry Medical College (1970).

Whipple, Alan (Allen) Oldfather (1881–1963). American surgeon. Developed procedure for resection of the pancreas (pancreaticoduodenectomy) known as the Whipple procedure. He was also known for developing the diagnostic triad for insulinoma known as Whipple's triad.

Wilder, Burt Green (1862–1925). American anatomist. Author of *What Young People*

Should Know, 1874; *Anatomical Technology*, 1882; *Physiology Practicums Emergences*, 1888; *Healthy Notes for Students*, 1890; *Brain of the Sheep*, 1903.

Wilkins, Maurice H. F. (1916–2004). New Zealand biochemist. Nobel laureate in Medicine or Physiology, 1962 (with F. H. C. Crick and J. D. Watson); proposed model for double-helix structure of DNA.

Williams, Daniel Hale (1856–1931). American surgeon. Pioneering heart surgeon; first physician to successfully perform open heart surgery in 1893. Contributed to health care for urban blacks in Chicago. Founder of Provident Hospital and Medical Center.

Wilson, Woodrow (1856–1924). 28th president of the United States of America (1913–1921)

Woodson, Carter G. (1875–1950). American historian and educator. Known as father of black history. Founded the Association for the Study of Negro Life and History (now the Association for the Study of African American Life and History) in 1915; founded *Journal of Negro History*; established Negro History Week (now Black History Month).

Wright, Louis Tompkins (1891–1952). American surgeon. First African American to get an M.D. degree from Harvard Medical School (1915). Invented the intradermal method of vaccination for smallpox. Wrote a section on skull fracture for Charles L. Scudder's *The Treatment of Fractures*, successfully challenging traditional theories on the treatment of such cases. Devised a blade plate for the operative treatment of fractures of the knee joint and a brace for cervical vertebrae fractures. For his noted work in surgery, admitted in 1934 to fellowship in the American College of Surgeons. Authority on head injury. President of the Harlem Medical Board. Pioneered studies of cancer chemotherapy. Successfully used aureomycin in humans. Conscientious crusader for equal rights for African Americans. Published 89 research articles.

Wylie, Ida Alexa Ross (1885–1959). Australian-born British writer. Published more than 30 books including *The Daughter of Braham* (1912); *Toward Morning* (1920); *The Silver Virgin* (1929); *To the Vanquished* (1934); *Furious Young Man* (1935); *A Feather in Her Hat* (1937); and *My Life with George* (1940).

Zacharias, Jerrold Reinach (1905–1986). American physicist. Researched atomic clocks, molecular beam magnetic resonance, and electric shape of atomic nuclei.

Zinsser, Hans (1878–1940). American bacteriologist. Author of *Rats, Lice and History* (1935). Researched cholera and other bacteriological diseases. Developed immunizations against typhus fever.

Zola, Emile (1840–1902). Renowned French novelist and critic. Founder of the Naturalist movement in literature.

Index